MOTHER'S SECRET

A Nutritionist's View of Family and Alzheimer's Disease

By
Marilyn Walls

Mother's Secret:
A Nutritionist's View of Family
and Alzheimer's Disease

ISBN: 978-0-9990792-0-1

This book is for my sisters, Beverly and Judy.
Together we loved and cared for Mother.

"My mother never really wanted to be filmed. When she got diagnosed with Alzheimer's she wanted to hide it.
I think that footage absolutely shows how much I love my mother.
And yet is absolutely a betrayal of her."

Kristen Johnson, documentarian,
from *Talk of the Town,* The New Yorker

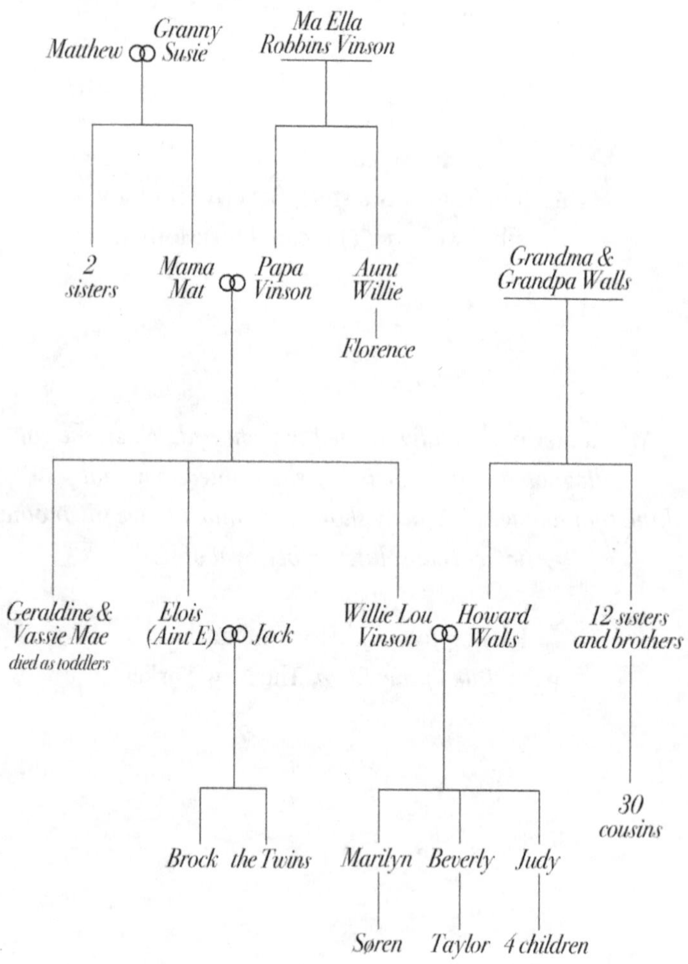

Matthew
Granny Susie
Ma Ella Robbins Vinson
2 sisters
Mama Mat
Papa Vinson
Aunt Willie
Florence
Grandma & Grandpa Walls
Geraldine & Vassie Mae
died as toddlers
Elois (Aint E)
Jack
Willie Lou Vinson
Howard Walls
12 sisters and brothers
Brock
the Twins
Marilyn
Beverly
Judy
30 cousins
Søren
Taylor
4 children

PROLOGUE

"Miz Walls. Miz Walls!" The stocky nurse in blue scrubs sternly demanded Mother's attention.

Mother stared with eyes as vacant as the church sanctuary following the final benediction. She turned her head, her white hair a wispy cloud cover in the anemic February grayness.

"Miz Walls!" The nurse persisted with her routine questions to check Mother's acuity. "Do you know where you are?"

Mother looked around the hygienic room, puzzled by the institutional box. She glanced at her daughters sitting on the narrow couch, where one of them would sleep each night.

The nurse urged. "Where are you?"

With a burst of cordiality reserved for preachers and Sam's Club greeters, Mother replied, "Right here."

The nurse pointed to us, Mother's daughters. "Who are they?"

To this query my clever mother manipulated, "Y'all introduce yourself."

We all laughed. Pleased, Mother looked at my sisters and me, who had given her grandchildren. "Are y'all in high school?"

The nurse continued, pointing to me, the eldest daughter. "Who's that?"

"A friend. We go waaaaay back."

The nurse patted the shoulder of Mother's middle daughter sitting in a chair next to the hospital bed. "And who's that"

Mother fondly put her hand on her daughter's platinum hair. "She's mine."

"What's her name?"

Mother smiled. "My love."

No one wants it: the doctor's slight frown and the tiny pitying look that precede the softly spoken curse, Alzheimer's disease. Medical science knows a lot about keeping many common diseases from killing us but very little about dealing with the breakdown of brain functioning. In fact, Alzheimer's is the only disease in the top ten with no prevention and no cure.

Dr. Alois Alzheimer discovered this dreadful disease in 1906 in Germany. A 51-year-old woman with unusual symptoms was brought to the psychiatric hospital. She told Dr. Alzheimer, "I've lost myself." After her death the doctor autopsied her brain and found "something sticky and starchy" along with twisted fibers. Thus began medical knowledge of this complex ailment. And over a hundred years later, Alzheimer's and aging continue to be confounding issues, a condition where both the patient and family lose themselves.

Alzheimer's disease (AD) might be considered an epidemic. These numbers from the Alzheimer's Association are frightening: over five million Americans currently have AD, and the cost of care exceeds $100 billion annually. One hundred thousand people in the U.S. die every year from AD. When the baby boomers become a part of these predictions, the entire federal budget could be consumed by taking care of those with this disease. With such dire numbers, many families will be beaten by these odds. My family was. Our mother became a statistic in these burgeoning Alzheimer's numbers.

This hybrid book offers a confluence of personal events and relevant information about Mother's descent into dementia. Think of the chapters as a rhythm, alternating science and memoir. Perhaps our experiences juxtoposed beside scientific knowledge will lend needed support to anyone facing these dilemmas. When I look back with the perfection of hindsight and I know the outcome of Mother's battle with Alzheimer's disease, what we did <u>not</u> do might appear obvious, even glaring. This all happened to us before the ready access of a Smart Phone in every pocket; no quick answers appeared on a colorful touch screen in our old-school world of the previous decade. Still the problems remain, all too similar, and the questions loom despite technological advances.

Another aspiration in writing this book is to protect our children from these hardships by preparing ourselves to grow older. Soon my generation will be the elders, faced with our own health issues and imminent deaths. My prayers requested a mystical "pound of prevention" in these pages: because this book is about <u>our</u> future, as well as about the present predicaments with our elders. Our consciousness and preparation can serve those who will be responsible for us during those last years.

Chapter 1

MISSISSIPPI ROOTS

"Mississippi is a place and a state of mind. The name evokes strong reactions from those who live here and from those who do not, but who think they know something about its people and their past."

Dennis Mitchell, A New History of Mississippi

As an impressionable twenty-something in the 1970s, far from my parents' house, I was living in Minnesota, a freezing winter land populated, appropriately, by Swedes and other Scandinavians. My new friends knew exactly which great-great-great aunt came around the world with her woolen scarves packed in her favorite dresser, which was, no doubt, still in their family. They asked me about my heritage, wondering where Southerners originated. I phoned my parents in Memphis, Tennessee, a city known more for Elvis than my family's accomplishments, and posed the question of my ancestry. I paused, expectantly, awaiting some grand narrative about my bloodlines.

My mother Lou responded, "Why, we're from Mis'sippi."

I pressed her, thinking she had missed the sweeping scope of my inquiry. "No, I mean are we French or English or Irish?"

"Why, we're just country people."

What a disappointment for me to be saddled with such a drab birthright. No migration stories across Europe, no Danish plates handed down through the generations, no china cabinets shipped with my kin to the New World. I was limited to a small radius of Mississippi, the poorest state in the union.

World War II brought many northern Mississippians into Memphis, the city on the bluff. For my parents, Lou and Howard Walls, who joined the Christian diaspora separately, it was a move of only a hundred miles. A hundred miles of dirt roads, driving on flimsy tires bought with World War II ration coupons, and a terrifying trek if you traced your roots only as far as Mis'sipi. My parents were a generation in transition, escaping the unpredictable crops and cows in a dust cloud dream of better jobs and more money. They lived in Me'fis with their livelihoods coming from new directions, while their parents, sisters, brothers and taste buds stayed behind on the farm. The crimson clay of their youth clung to them as to Eudora Welty's fiction.

My progenitors hailed from scruffy backwoods. In the vicinity of Algoma, my father, Howard Walls, grew up surrounded by impoverished farmland and "dirt-poor" relatives. My mother, born as Willie Lou Vinson to Mama Mat and Papa Vinson, came from dots along dusty Mississippi byways, Guntown and Blue Springs. There she and her only surviving sister Elois, who in southern speak was Aint E to my sisters and me, played on tire swings until they were old enough to help out in the Vinson family business, a true mom-and-pop country store with light slanting up through the plank floorboards.

Those Vinsons were salt of the earth folks. They didn't drink, though Papa Vinson, tall and gaunt with hallow cheeks, smoked unfiltered cigarettes. Mama Mat, her real name Mattie after her father Matthew, was tiny without an ounce of fat. She dipped Garrett's Snuff, spitting the dark residue into a canning jar hidden beside her bed. Though small, Mama Mat could grab a chicken, wring its neck with one tiny hand, chop off its head on the tree stump, be undeterred as the headless chicken ran around crazily, and fry up the plucked pieces for lunch, the grease from each breaded morsel soaking into a dish towel on a chipped plate.

Working hard must have developed as a genetic survival requirement from lifetimes of Mississippi farming. However, as a child Mother was protected from the worst of that life. In the sizzling summers of the 1920s Deep South she played barefoot in the dirt, a tall child with brown hair chopped short, wearing a homemade dress with a big white collar. She was the favorite of the neighbor women.

"Why do you say I'm spoiled?" Mother, charming from a young age, asked Miz Rosabell, who lived down the road from the Vinsons and petted little Willie Lou.

"You aren't spoiled," Miz Rosabell teased her. "You're tainted!"

Mother knew tainted was even worse, like bad meat kept too long in the smoke house, and it would make you sick if you ate it. "But you said I'm so sweet I might melt when it rains."

Miz Rosabell kissed little Lou on the top of her head, "You're both."

At five years old, my precocious mother snuck prematurely into the first grade where Miz Rosabell was the teacher. It was in the new school building, right across the road from home, where her father—Papa Vinson to me—was the principal. Schools depended on community involvement, and Papa Vinson had helped raise the money for this new building, which expanded from a three-room school to a four-teacher school with an auditorium. At about thirty years old with only an eighth-grade education, Papa Vinson had gone every week to Normal School to become certified as a teacher, leaving his wife—my grandmother Mama Mat -- with the babies and the farm. Normal Schools, which trained teachers and later became teachers' colleges, started in the seventeenth century in France, spread throughout Europe, and reached the U.S. in 1839. They were finally founded, fifty-five years later, in Mississippi in 1896, three decades after the Civil War had ended. In the twenty-nine years of the existence of Normal Schools in the state of Mississippi, Papa Vinson was student number 296 to receive this certification because only an average of ten people annually completed the qualifications. This was the beginning of education as the touchstone of Papa Vinson's family; even during the Depression he sent both of his daughters to college by cashing in his life insurance policy. The sacrifices netted benefits; the Vinsons settled into Cedar Hill, no longer living as renters, and they had their own store with Papa Vinson listed as a "merchant" in the 1930 census.

Families, when my mother Lou was a child, were unable to get together that often, as travel was too difficult. Once my aunt Elois--Mother's big sister--explained to me, matter-of-factly, in her whispery voice, "We didn't have parties." The Vinsons did, however, have someone living with them most of the time. A grandmother or some aunt, bereaved women and children in the precarious years before Social Security, or a lone bachelor returned to the farm after a stint on a Mississippi River barge. Since Papa Vinson extended credit to his neighbors when supplies and food were needed from his store, I assume he was a pillar of their rural community. That, however, did not make Papa Vinson rich. He took promissory notes in exchange for supplies, payment to come with the harvest. In those grim times it must have been a necessary risk of doing business, since many of those promises could not be kept.

The Vinsons went to church. Mama Mat was in the choir, singing on the church lawn on Sunday afternoons, hymns shaped by pointed, triangular notes and twangy harmony. The neighbors came for quiltings, to slaughter a hog, and to sit on an upturned barrel on the porch of Papa Vinson's store. There were extra folks at every Vinson supper. It wasn't a party, but it was, like the daily rites of endurance, communal.

Mother knew the high expectations associated with public responsibility. In contrast, Daddy's family was acquainted with hunger and poverty.

Daddy was the third of thirteen Walls brothers and sisters, born in 1912 in a two-room house in Pontotoc County, Mississippi. Too poor even to be affected by the Depression, the Walls were loud and bold, compensating for scarcity with outrageousness. They learned to enliven the hard times with a sense of humor and irrepressible determination. Those old clichés were Daddy's realities: after sleeping in one bed with four or five of his siblings, he brought in the wood on cold winter mornings to start the fire. When he and his brothers and sisters weren't working in the fields, they walked five miles in the worst of weather to a one-room schoolhouse. They knew the trials of working among the scrawny cotton plants. As a teen-ager Daddy was plowing cotton when a mule kicked one of his younger sisters in the head. Daddy took his sobbing little sister on his back, carrying her up and down though the ditches and gullies to get help. Later when he left the farm and moved to Memphis, he sent that same sister $1 every week for her own escape.

Great-great-great grandfather Walls kept fighting after The War Between the States was over. That mule-headedness seethed into the extreme deprivations visited on great-great-great-grandfather Walls' descendants, crusting them in the temptations and deep companionship associated with such destitution.

When Daddy, along with most of his siblings, and a cousin or two were all living together at the "home place" in Algoma, Grandma Walls--Daddy's mother--fed all those mouths with biscuits. Sometimes those biscuits enfolded sausage or fried ham from a hog that had been killed and dressed, but at other times there was simply jelly from the small apples in the orchard or sorghum molasses. Only special occasions merited the sacrifice of the oldest hen, one too aged to secure her existence by laying eggs for a needy family. One night after a supper of biscuits and sausage gravy, the dishes washed in water from the pump, Grandma Walls looked down the road at a lone figure walking toward their house. It was Dewey, one of her seven younger brothers; those brothers, scheming their way out of white trash dregs, became sharp dressers, always with a cocked hat and shined shoes.

Putting the handkerchief, which she always clutched tightly, into her apron pocket and straightening a plain dress on her plump, baby-making body, Grandma Walls said to her daughter Alma, "What're we gonna feed Dewey? Ya know he ain't eaten. I just got enough food for breakfast, but if I make supper for Dewey, we won't have nothin' left."

However, a dearth of ingredients never stopped Grandma Walls from shaking out the last of her flour and feeding hungry family. Dewey sat on the bench beside the long table, kidded with his nephews, and appreciatively ate the meal that Grandma Walls cooked for him. He headed back down the road later that night, kicking up coin-sized gravel with his flashy shoes to ward off the bright-eyed creatures lurking in the country bush. When Grandma Walls, cleaning up one more time, took a rag to the flour bin, she found a twenty-dollar bill hidden underneath.

"Look what Dewey left!" Grandma Walls exclaimed. "That'll feed us for a whole month. I reckon I aughta feel bad, cause ya know this is ill-gotten gain." Dewey, like several of Grandma Walls' brothers, was a gambler and a con man. But there was something of a Biblical blessing in the biscuits she threw out on the rough family waters coming back to her twenty-fold.

My parents met in Memphis during World War II. They had grown up within twenty-five miles of each other, though worlds apart in many ways. Swept away by the glorious attraction of opposites, they fell in love and married. Lou and Howard were an amazing team. After all, it took a like-minded and clever partner to stretch the budget when Howard would go and bail an employee out of jail, to cook for all the lonely college students he would bring home from church, and to do all the office work while he kept the business growing.

My sisters, Beverly and Judy, and I were baby boomers, and the number of our first cousins added to that much-chronicled population explosion, especially from Daddy's Walls siblings: thirteen brothers and sisters begat nearly thirty-five cousins. Regularly when my sisters and I were kids, our family drove for two hours south from Memphis to Mississippi to visit our relatives, to bring back freshly butchered beef, and always, always, always for holidays, the trunk of the car loaded with carefully wrapped Mother's Day presents or homemade cakes stashed in Tupperware. Nothing in our city life compared to being with our Mississippi cousins. In our sheltered Memphis neighborhood where we went to church with most of the people who lived on our street, Mother ruled our life with strict boundaries: stay in the backyard, don't ride your bike past that first telephone pole, don't go into the next-door neighbor's house. But in Mis'sippi, Mother relaxed her grip, her panic for our safety assuaged by the native grounds of her own childhood. Gardens, pastures, and cotton fields stretched every which-a-way at both grandparental farms; and at the edge of a wide front yard was a bumpy, gravel road. A distant dust cloud might signal the truck coming down the road to collect the dented milk cans, full from the dawn milking. We'd make guesses at the dust trail, waiting for the far-away noise of the engine to distinguish itself as a pickup or a tractor. We swung on ropes across gullies, swam in creeks brown with mud, and spent hours making up games and contests beside the giant oak tree, alive with legends of Confederate sharp shooters tucked in the upper branches. In the ebony country nights, we hid behind the hen house or deep in the garden foliage during courageous games of Kick the Can. On Christmas Eve we emblazoned the black as coal sky with dazzling and dangerous fireworks.

Mama Mat and Papa Vinson's "li'l store," with a Quaker State gas pump and a big red "Drink Coca-Cola" sign, was right across the rural road from their white asbestos-shingled house, but we kids had to ask permission to go there. Papa Vinson would amble across the sun-parched front yard, wearing a tight-lipped solemnity and his straw fedora that left a horizontal tan line bisecting his forehead. He would nod to us kids who played under the shade of the massive oak tree, three boy cousins and the three Memphis sisters, address us collectively and individually as "boy" or "girl," then cross the dusty road to the li'l store. Sometimes, though, he would give us coins to spend and lead the six of us over the red gravel like a gaggle of baby geese, honking excitedly behind his silent stride. I would take my prized dime and buy a Three Musketeers bar, the chocolate white with age, and we would weigh our growing bodies on the scale that also told our fortune. "Somebody loves you." Those fortunes were mostly disappointments, compared to our bigger dreams. Sometimes Papa Vinson took us fishing at the pond on the other side of the pasture. We all sat on the dirt beside the cloudy water with bamboo fishing poles; for the scaredy cats Papa Vinson would bait hooks with wiggling worms. It was the same pond, much to our dismay, where bags of wild barn kittens met the end of their extremely short existences. We grandkids knew Papa Vinson was Justice of the Peace (JP), an elected local official, and that he had big leather-bound books titled in gold as a part of that job. He could marry people but usually sent the eager couples on down the road to Brother Rakestraw, the Baptist preacher. The rest of Papa Vinson's JP duties did not interest us cousins. Neither did we care that he was a director of the Federal Land Bank, a state duty that took him as far as Illinois. A 1956 article in the local newspaper about his bountiful farming techniques opened with "D.L. Vinson, president of the Union County Farm Bureau, has developed a successful 183-acre dairy and row-crop farm on the once-eroded hill land in the Ellistown community." Decades after his death I learned about sustainable farming and biodiversity, and then understood the scope of his agricultural acumen and his dedication to the land. As kids we saw him merely as our taciturn grandfather, lanky and skinny in his overalls, his tractor a speck on the other side of the pastures, the deep crimson clover blossoms surreally separating him from our games. To entertain us while Mother, Mama Mat and Aint E were still in the kitchen putting leftovers in the oven and washing dishes, Papa Vinson would bring us the much anticipated treat at the end of a carefree summer day: a juicy red watermelon to drip sticky on our bare legs. City manners did not keep us girls from competing in the watermelon seed spitting contests, but Aint E's three boys, who had to go to un-air conditioned school in sweaty July because Mississippi kids needed to pick cotton in the fall, always won.

In our June Cleaver world of black and white television sitcoms, mothers called themselves homemakers and fathers often ran a small business. School, church, our friends, Memphis State University and Daddy's business were only about a mile from our house. Though Daddy's business was blue collar, we never realized that, as it was a part of the Highland community: a neighborhood of other family-owned businesses. We knew the owners of the grocery store (went to high school with his sons), the bakery (same church), the drug store (coke floats and cheap eau de cologne), the café (greasy lunch), the dairy queen (banana splits after church on Sunday night) and the jewelry store (necklaces that exceeded our Christmas budgets). Daddy was on the board to build the new Highland branch YMCA, our doctors were around the corner, we got books from the public library, and, of course, loved to shop at the "5 and dime" store. Being Memphis, a plethora of church steeples graced the neighborhood.

Daddy, wearing service station coveralls, a glimpse of disco jumpsuits to come, was the boss at "the place." His corner included an Esso station, a state-of-the-art automotive garage, with a parts department. The prerequisite "white only" restrooms and drinking fountains were in the front, with the "colored" relegated embarrassingly to the back. We waited endless hours for Daddy to disengage from customers or employees, Mother impatient that we would again be arriving late. My sisters and I passed the time trying to make the bell inside the service station ring when we jumped on that hose that spanned the asphalt. That bell alerted that customers had arrived to have gas pumped, windshields cleaned, and tires and oil checked. Eventually Daddy also sold pop-up camping trailers there, bragging that his daughters could put the camper up in record-breaking time. His watch in hand, he actually timed us on our camping trips to the cliffs and lakes of nearby state parks.

In Me'fis our plates were loaded with Mis'sipi vegetables. Each summer Mother said to Daddy, "Mama called today. The beans (or corn or tomatoes or okra) are ready." The next day Mother packed us girls into the fin-tailed Oldsmobile, leaving Daddy at work. Once again we crossed the state line. Soon we begged Mother to speed up on Bunk'um Hill, a roller coaster (to us) stretch of bumpy road just before we arrived at the farm. However, much to our disappointment those sweltering summer afternoons, Mother declined our need for gravel road excitement, Daddy being looser with the accelerator on Mississippi curves. That night we slept with the windows open, and before we woke the next morning to the greetings of roosters and cows, to the smell of hay and heat, Mama Mat and Mother were already in the garden with big straw hats and bushel baskets. While we girls were spared the prickly garden, not adept enough to leave flat beans on the vine, we had the unrelenting job of shelling those freshly picked beans.

We refined an expertise in the art of shelling speckled butter beans. First, pull the vein, which once connected the bean to the stalk, to loosen the pod. With a swift thumb action open the pod and plop the hard, fat beans into a bowl or shoebox, whichever we were assigned. Before long our thumbnails were green, and the contents of our bowls or shoeboxes were contributed into the kitchen sink, where Mama Mat and Mother washed our wares. They packed little plastic bags into cardboard freezer boxes, each full of fresh gifts from the garden and hand labeled with the vegetable name and date. Though Mother proudly announced the daily count of "quarts of butter beans put up," the designated shellers became more irritable as the full bushel baskets heavy with the garden harvests continued to multiply. Contests were invented, money was proffered on both a piecework and hourly basis, and when all else failed, orders and threats prevailed over our whining and fussing. Purple hull peas were easier: those little round numbers fairly leapt out of their pods, while string beans made crisp snaps as we segmented them. The endless supply of legumes loomed like a specter. Even on the way home in the car we filled our traveling shoeboxes, until we finished our requirements back in Memphis. During the winter Mother cajoled us when she took the beans out of the freezer and cooked them all day with a taste of bacon grease and sugar, "See, aren't these good? Aren't y'all glad for all that work y'all did?" What I wanted to say was "Sure, mom, my thumb is permanently fractured, we have eternal emotional band-aids from our arguments, and none of my friends are forced to eat four vegetables at each meal." But I didn't dare. Instead I cleaned my plate so I could have dessert. It's no wonder I eventually became a vegetarian.

The only difference between our mother and our friends' mothers, as my sisters and I saw it, was our mother did more and did it better. Her house, reflective of her life, was always in order. She cooked constantly, fed visiting missionaries, sewed most of our clothes, checked our homework nightly with a critical eye, made graceful flower arrangements for Garden Club, all the while watching our girlish behavior as a PTA room mother and the church maven. Our African-American maid, Nonie, who cleaned for us five days a week and ironed listening to her "stories" on the tall Philco radio in the hall, lightened Mother's load for $5 a day. Mother also worked at "the place" every week, doing bookkeeping and payroll for the twenty or so employees. She lived in the present, worried about the future, and never talked about the past.

I grew up in a time of unprecedented financial growth, of kids having more opportunities than their parents, of school honors, of advancement. And so our lives progressed, into bigger and better houses with more streamlined appliances, plusher furniture, flocked wallpaper, and a trampoline and ping-pong table. We took piano lessons, got a red and white motorboat and water-skied on sparkly mirror lakes; we camped in the Great Smoky Mountains. Life was thrilling.

Many of us boomer cousins did not allow our Mississippi origins to confine us. My two sisters and I moved our families along less volatile waterways across the country. My youngest sister Judy and her husband Buddy eventually settled in Chattanooga, via Ohio and China, their four offspring grown into young adults on their own. Bev, her husband Mitchell, and their daughter Taylor lived in northern California. I was in Seattle while my son Søren pursued his academic ambitions through various universities. As we spread out across the continent, even the allure of holidays did not bring us all together. The dirt roads of our past were widened and paved, smooth blacktop concealing those magical journeys of long ago.

After almost forty-five years of marriage, Daddy died of pancreatic cancer in 1990. Mother learned to live alone. She managed so well that I kidded her that she was the poster child for widowhood. We were all proud of her independence and decision-making. She consulted us on none of her choices. She sold her columned, colonial-style house and bought a condominium by a golf course in the suburbs. It all worked fine, until it didn't. By then the patterns had been established, and Mother and her daughters were in trouble.

Chapter 2

THE SCIENCE OF A THOUSAND SUBTRACTIONS

> *"No matter who you are, what you've accomplished, what your financial situation is - when you're dealing with a parent with Alzheimer's, you yourself feel helpless. As the disease unfolds, you don't know what to expect."*
>
> *Maria Shriver*

In a country top-heavy with the elderly, the uncertainties about an aging parent can dominate. Rather than dinner party banter, the conversations may bemoan an ailing mother, the ambulance to the emergency room or the fight to move a defiant parent to assisted living. My sisters and I reflected this uncomfortable trend as we grappled with Mother's behavior. As a smear on the larger canvas of aging demographics, my color palate blended into the perplexing new pattern of caregiving. Born into a generation refusing to be confined, I rebelled against my elders. I married, divorced, went to graduate school, took jobs in other states, and joined the mobile society, climbing corporate ladders and leaving my parents behind. Strange, then, to be confronted with parents as they aged and died, to be responsible for decisions parents did not trust us, their adult offspring, to make.

As a parent's behavior changes, their children desire clarifications. Seeking to understand Mother's growing negativism, I summoned the facts of how synapses become patterned over time. Feelings and attitudes have synaptic pathways. We feel happy and certain synapses fire. Over time this synaptic corridor becomes like a brain rut. This could lead to a younger testy person becoming especially cantankerous in old age. On the other hand, greasing those positive synapses with repetition early in life might pay off with a more optimistic outlook as an elder. The power of positive thinking: maybe it's basic brain chemistry or a neuronal blueprint. When Mother would get mad, my sisters and I would think, "She's always been tough to please. Maybe it's just a brain habit gone bad." We thought by convincing Mother to look on the bright side, to fight her entrenched critical nature, that we could change the situation. Little did we know we were suggesting logic to a brain gone amuck. We could not admit it might be Alzheimer's disease.

MENTAL LOSSES

The first clues of Alzheimer's disease (AD) are naturally the noticeable symptoms exhibited by the patient. Unfortunately, deterioration in critical areas of the brain may precede symptoms by many years, perhaps even ten to twenty.[1] "No impairment" has been described as Stage 1 of Alzheimer's disease; the person appears normal while the brain bit by bit, neuron by neuron, silently loses functionality. Symptoms, therefore, may be gradual and insidious, possibly appearing to be behavior patterns, simply neurons in a rut, which are accepted over time as personality traits. The symptoms of this degenerative disease might get labeled incorrectly as bitchiness or crankiness. The individual gets "blamed" for the behavior rather than the family acknowledging the disease. Family stories get retrieved. Hasn't she always been a little hysterical? Remember how hardheaded she was.

The first admitted symptom of Alzheimer's is most often forgetfulness. This forgetfulness may be diagnosed as mild cognitive impairment (MCI). The biological changes in the brain of someone with MCI are identical with the mess in an Alzheimer's-affected brain.[2] There is deficient memory with MCI, and the problems with language or other essential cognitive functions are severe enough to be noticed by others. The changes can even be reflected on cognitive tests. What buttresses the person with MCI is the ability to handle these mental roadblocks so that they do not especially interfere with daily life. [3]

Though MCI carries an increased risk of developing AD, not everyone with MCI progresses to AD. A 2013 review of 14 studies considering the conversion of MCI to Alzheimer's disease found 5.4% - 16.5% of participants progressed annually to Alzheimer's dementia.[4] Simple math, therefore, supports a glass half full for some with MCI. While experts may think of MCI as the intermediate stage between normal aging and AD, it remains a mystery why some MCI patients can live out their lives remaining stable or on occasion even return to normal. During MCI there is still hope for treatment and for delaying the symptoms. MCI symptoms indicate a need to stop and evaluate, get thee to a doctor, show the kids where all the bank accounts are, take steps to turn down the stress, and turn up the exercise.

Memory loss, especially short term, is a prominent warning sign of AD as well as MCI. David Shenk, author of "The Forgetting," describes having Alzheimer's disease as a person who is the sum of memories, evaporating in the slow "death of a thousand subtractions."[5] Long-term memory is stored differently in the brain than short-term memory and protected from early deterioration. Many older people have had what is laughingly called a "senior moment;" thus, forgetfulness is automatically associated with aging. This in itself is fraught with difficulty. Such symptoms can be caused by something other than Alzheimer's. Memory loss and behavior issues can be caused by a series of minor strokes, fluid on the brain, small blood clots in vessels supplying the brain, a brain tumor, depression, female urinary tract infections, hypothyroidism, drug reactions, or poor nutrition. Obviously, some of those causes are fixable. What family member or elder wouldn't want to believe that a pill for a urinary tract condition holds the solution? Hence, out of fear or reality, it is easy to be deluded about Alzheimer's. Therefore, it is often after a process of elimination and many tests that Alzheimer's is diagnosed.

In the beginning it starts slowly, the protein clumps cause plaques, clog up the brain, get in the way of the neurons, then stop the synapses. It is all about those brain pathways, about the neurons and their ability to connect, to "talk" to one another. Neurons communicate by sending messages with electrical brain charges and chemicals called neurotransmitters. AD destroys neurons; as these neurons become unable to function, they die. The brain shrinks, losing volume quickly, and the loss of volume is a "markedly accelerated atrophy rate compared to non-demented individuals."[6] A most complicated muscle atrophy. Millions of synapses dissolve as brain cells die, causing the shrinkage. This brain atrophy correlates with neuronal loss and leads to dementia. The good news is that the brain has plenty of back up in its network in the early stages. During this initial synapse loss, there are still neighboring cells healthy enough to pick up the slack.[7] Other brain regions compensate for the non-functioning areas, basically doing brain tasks not really their job. These cognitive reserves come from multiple sources and are not likely a fixed entity, because the brain both passively and actively attempts to cope with changes and pathology.[8] How these reserves were established is one of the many conundrums of AD. Whether from education, lifestyle choices or some unknown factor, the yet-to-be patient has reserves to make up for the memory slips or to keep it together when daughters visit.

Is there a way to nurture the brain's ability to make up for this cell loss? A study scored 1157 people, 65 years plus, according to their participation in brain stimulating activities. Those who kept busy learning something new as they aged and who engaged regularly in mentally stimulating activities had higher cognitive test scores. Ten years later all these people were revisited. For those who maintained mental activities and also developed dementia, it was found that their time without symptoms was extended, and when the decline began, it was much faster than the decline of those who were not mentally active. The study theorized that mentally engaged people build up a cognitive reserve that may help them compensate when the initial brain changes associated with dementia and Alzheimer's begin to develop.[9] Therefore, when those symptoms did surface, the physical and mental deterioration happened much faster. The slope was steep, an out-of-control sled on an icy hill. The speedy declivity was a blessing, nonetheless, because patients spent a shorter time with the disease affecting their lives. Neither did they suffer as long at the end of their lives compared to those not mentally active. The experts believe that the brain was able to compensate longer with the mental resources created by new learning activities.[10]

The challenge for the brain is to try something different, to take on a frustrating task because it forces neurotransmitters into alternate paths. Even someone who does crossword puzzles daily could benefit by learning to quilt or focusing on a skill that pushes the brain's comfort zones. That explanation could have been an answer to my despair, "How did Mother get so bad in such a short time?" She had been a mentally involved person. Those same kinds of neuronal reserves assisted our mother with her "Great Cover-up." However, the cycle of destruction, the flood of sticky globs, and the unexplained tangles in the brain circuitry eventually became like kudzu, that climbing, coiling, and trailing vine so invasive in Mother's native Mississippi.

Having grown up in the south, I've seen kudzu engulf the gentle hillsides, seen it tenting trees. My cousin Brock told me it grew three feet a day, while the myth persists that the kudzu plant grows a mile a minute. Though Willie Morris called kudzu "sinister," kudzu was brought from Japan to heal the land after "decades of careless cotton and tobacco farming had depleted Southern soil and bankrupt farmers were fleeing their barren fields."[11] Kudzu literally took over the landscape, making it a fitting metaphor for Alzheimer's disease choking off the workings of the brain.

It is heart-breaking, this AD inability to convert thoughts to pen or voice, to see all the effort required to conserve that precious skill of communication, long accepted as normal, as a basic human right. In a major misinterpretation of our mother's problems, we faulted her poor hearing for her difficulty talking on the phone. All she needed was a new hearing aid. Mother, too, thought a better hearing aid would solve her communication difficulties. It seems apparent in retrospect that Alzheimer's was causing her problems with talking on the phone. It takes time for someone with AD to process thoughts and conversation, to dig through the cerebral kudzu and find those cognitive reserves. They also need visual cues. But we did not know that abrupt changes in conversation were difficult for Mother to anticipate and follow, did not realize it was her comprehension that suffered. We thought she could not hear us; it was far worse than that. She was not able to grasp what we were saying. And by the time she had sloughed through the mental undergrowth, her impatient daughters had moved on in the conversation or made her angry by verbally discarding what she did unearth.

PHYSICAL CHANGES

Physical dysfunction such as falling may be the first true but unrecognized symptoms of this disease. Physical symptoms like falling and balance problems may exhibit at the onset of Alzheimer's disease before mental symptoms. A study of elders led by Susan Stark at Washington University School of Medicine in St. Louis showed that there were almost twice as many falls in those with plaque build-up but no cognitive impairment compared to those with low levels of plaque. If there was evident cognitive impairment, earlier studies had already found that fall risk was "substantially increased." Thus, the more brain plaques, the more risk of falls, whether or not there are cognitive symptoms.[12]

Alzheimer's causes visual and spatial issues, like trouble distinguishing the relationship between the body and objects around the body. Perhaps the patient cannot tell where the wall ends and the floor starts due to loss of visual acuity. This can include a deficit in distinguishing color, contrast or visual fields, but often cannot be diagnosed by a regular eye exam.[13] Since an AD patient probably cannot explain this, poor eyesight or other bodily frailties are cited for these misperceptions, these trip-ups. According to her unsuspecting daughters, what Mother needed was an eye exam and new glasses.

Then as Alzheimer's progresses, other symptoms appear: disorientation, dysphasia (an inability to find the right word), and sudden, unpredictable mood swings. In the later stages there can be severe confusion, even hallucinations and delusions, wandering, incontinence, loss of bowel control, and neglect of personal hygiene. Eventually the patient must be given medications by others, can no longer handle money or finances, does not understand what people are saying, has given up reading, and has problems with writing (or can no longer write). Speech becomes unintelligible. The list is long and devastating: agitation, anxiety, apathy, disinhibition, irritability, repetitive motor disturbances, sleep disruptions, and changes in eating.

DIAGNOSING ALZHEIMER'S DISEASE

Given this disturbing array of misplaced indictment, how does one find answers about the abilities of a mentally weakening elder? Since Alzheimer's disease has been studied for decades, there are a variety of cognitive tests helpful for identifying features and markers of this dreaded malady. Neurologists or physicians can administer tests that indicate a patient's mental troubles. One of these tests is the Clinical Dementia Rating (CDR). The CDR offers a scale of cognitive and functional performance in six areas. The MSSI is another cognitive assessment tool used by doctors during an office visit to detect mental impairment. Often a series of tests validate the diagnosis of Alzheimer's disease. A clinical neuropsychologist can be trained to differentiate between normal changes in memory that occur with aging, isolated memory problems that do not constitute dementia, and a range of patterns that are associated with the different dementias. Other tests distinguish between depression and dementia. These are the tests that Mother resisted, the doctors' appointments we would make in the future as denial lost its stronghold, the appointments she would cancel.

Not long ago the medical reality was that there were no physical lab tests to verify an Alzheimer's diagnosis. When Mother was symptomatic, not that long ago, testing for AD was impossible. The only definitive diagnosis was by looking at brain tissue, either during an autopsy or a biopsy. This is still the best verification. Brain atrophy that can be seen on an MRI is not present until much later stages of AD; by the time it is visible on an MRI, a diagnosis is not going to make any difference.

However, new research is changing the arena of identification and some of these new methods are being used in medical studies. At this time these procedures are very expensive and probably not available for most people. Biomarkers of proteins can be measured in the cerebral spinal fluid. New discoveries are happening at a rapid pace. At the University of Pittsburgh cutting edge experiments are taking place. There the Pittsburgh Compound B stain (PiB) was developed; with a functional MRI and positron emission tomography, the compound B stains and highlights the amyloid plaques. This technique can be useful in showing amyloid levels, even when a person is asymptomatic.[14] Other advances and projects can be found on the website of Washington University's "Alzheimer's Disease and Research Center." This is a constantly evolving field, and what is known today might be usurped tomorrow.

AD SYMPTOMS AND STAGES

While AD progression is fluid and individual, a slope of hills and valleys rather than an immediate descent, stages can be identified. This list was complied from a variety of books and Internet sites, which are cited in the back of the book.

MILD

Memory loss, trouble recalling what happened recently

Confusion, getting lost in familiar settings, wandering

Organizational difficulties, poor judgment

Placing items in odd places

Difficulty with daily tasks such as household chores, anything with multiple steps from recipes and planning meals to playing cards

May be aware of losing these abilities

Depression symptoms (sadness, loss of energy, decreased interest in usual activities).

Mood swings, distrust, more stubbornness, changes in personality, easily upset

Social withdrawal, avoiding usual interests (which may be caused by the frustration of recognizing the changes happening or as protection against these changes being noticed)

Restlessness, aggressiveness, anxiety

Problems taking meds

Problems with abstract thinking and sequencing

Trouble understanding visual images, spatial relationships, and judging distance

Trouble joining in conversations; problems with words or speaking, using the wrong name to identify objects

Relying on someone else, even a spouse, to make decisions or answer questions they would've previously handled themselves

MODERATE

More and worsening behavior problems

May no longer be able to cover up the problems and symptoms

More memory loss, loss of current information

Trouble remembering home address or personal phone number

Delusions (mistaken beliefs)

Continually repeating stories word for word, making up stories to fill in the memory gaps, repeating the same question over and over

Beginning to forget facts of the past

Confusion about current events, time, and place

Difficulty with checkbook, paying bills, shopping, and numbers

Lessening comprehension, trouble writing, reading, or even watching TV

Problems with bathroom habits, not showering

Sloppy table manners

More easily agitated, defensive, in denial

Vulnerable to scams

Repetitive movements (rocking, rubbing)

Paranoia, delusions, hallucinations

Diminishing intellect and reasoning

Lack of concern for appearance and hygiene, trouble choosing what to wear; wearing the same clothes and insisting the clothes are still clean

Disorientation and falls; gait or walking problems which affect mobility and coordination

SEVERE

Needs full-time care

Loss of verbal skills

Groaning, screaming, mumbling

Delirium

Difficulty walking

Cries out inappropriately

Refusal to eat

Failure to recognize faces, even family or caregivers

Bladder or bowel incontinence

Aprixial (can't perform physical tasks like eating or dressing)

Aphasia (loss of ability to comprehend written or spoken word)

Confusing past and present

Chapter 3

THE SIN OF DENIAL

"Something in us wishes to remain a child, to be unconscious...to reject everything strange, or to do nothing."
Carl Jung

Memphis, Christmas Holidays 2007

Mother squinted through smudged glasses, her face as tight as stitches on a prize-winning quilt. "You are not going to come in here and take over my life! I can take care of myself. I don't need you trying to boss me around."

"But you can't hear us on the phone. And you've had this hearing aid for years." I stepped into forbidden terrain, the daughter who "talked back." An attitude not allowed when I was sixteen and still taboo at sixty.

"I do NOT need to go to the hearing aid doctor!" Mother said, her usually flat syllables sharp with disdain. "And I will NOT wear one of those behind-the-ear hearing aids! They look awful." This declaration from my mother who had consistently renounced vanity on the backs of Biblical passages. Practical to a fault, eye shadow and mascara mattered little to her. Prayer rather than make-up luminesced her morning ritual. She straightened the stack of newspapers on the coffee table. "You don't know what I do. You don't live here. Why do you have to argue with me so much?"

"I'm not arguing. I'm just trying to help," I said, my victim perspective cornmeal-coated in self-pity.

She got up and marched into the kitchen. "You're outta line! Just stop it!"

"But you're the one arguing with me," I mouthed to myself, not moving from the pale love seat. "I was only trying to help," became my refrain, a hymn promising to wash my sins as white as snow.

Fracas rather than festivity decorated the Christmas season of 2007 that I spent at Mother's home in Memphis. We sat in the pastel abundance of an overstuffed room. The zigzag fabric of her couches reflected a southern orchard, the pillows sewn in matching Cling Peach tones. For over fifteen years after Daddy's death Mother lived independently in the city by the roiling Mississippi River. Other women in similar situations faltered, begged their kids for assistance, were unable to drive or to balance their checkbooks. Mother's decision-making skills had made my sisters and me proud, had lifted our daughterly load.

I blamed our current problems on the distance between my home in Seattle and Mother's in Memphis, a separation that concealed her daily failures and encouraged delusion about her abilities. Our respective freedoms had come to define us, single women, living alone. Proud of our competency, we each guarded our solitude and the right to do as we pleased. I believed that living in closer proximity would allow us the literal avenues for working through our disparate perspectives. While more regular contact might have presented opportunities for building relationships, aging also required letting go, something steadily resisted. Most difficult of all, roles must be reversed.

Denial ran deep in my genes, infiltrating several generations of ancestors and dating back to that great-great-great grandfather, an unrepentant Confederate guerilla in the Civil War who refused to surrender after General Lee had laid down his sword. In Carl Jung's philosophy, denial allowed the shadow self to hide. Uncertainty cast a cloud: was the shadow my fear about confronting Mother or was my dread about Mother's erratic behavior? Both Mother and I presumed a thousand explanations to elucidate her forgetfulness and factiousness, making us like Paul Harding's description in *tinkers*, "maybe our shadows are in cahoots, sweet pea; maybe they're partners in crime, just like us."

Growing up my sisters and I were not permitted to disagree with our parents, our opinions discouraged or ignored. Although Mother got mad at us, I never heard Mother and Daddy fight. If unpleasantness or gossip erupted, Daddy would flash his coy smile and say, "Isn't it a beeeauuutiful day?!" Our cue to change the subject. If we persisted, Daddy would quote Jiminy Cricket, "If ya cain't say somethin' nice, don't say nothin' at all." At those words we were programmed to look at the praise-worthy sunshine and suppress any hint of negativity. Thus, disputes were new territory for Mother and me, a lawless place with no protective Daddy and no Disneyland escapes.

For days Mother and I squabbled, moments of repose as sparse as the few Christmas decorations in her home. She asked me a question. I answered in my megaphone voice.

"What?" she glared at me.

I raised the decibel level one more turn of the radio dial.

"What?" she challenged.

I answered even louder.

She snapped. "Don't yell at me!"

Looking for simple answers, I thought I could right everything in a few days with a new hearing aid. Brain disturbances were not on my radar.

My son and only offspring Søren, working on his PhD in Cincinnati, joined Mother and me for Christmas that year in Memphis, his calm spirit a buffer for the few days he was with us. Poor Søren had his grandmother complaining in one ear about me while I bitched in his other ear about her. Mother and I disagreed about everything; driving directions, though, were our specialty, whether to go left or right required the difficult negotiations usually reserved for Mideast Peace conferences. To relieve those tensions, in the evening the three of us played progressive rummy, a card game famous in our family, dealt for decades on kitchen tables and in motor homes. We sat around a square card table, unfolded in the middle of the living room.

Mother struggled with her cards. "What is it I'm looking for?" she asked, as she placed several cards face down and frowned at the ones she kept in her hands.

I looked at Søren, raising my eyebrows; Mother couldn't make a simple book of matching numbers.

Søren leaned over and quietly took the correct cards from Mother's hand. "Look, you have a book of three's right here," he congratulated her, putting down her books and runs as well as his own throughout the game. She had helped Søren when his fingers were little and the playing cards too big, lining his cards up in the lid of an aluminum foil box, while Daddy slid Søren the right card to play. The grandkids always won in card games with my parents. Beautifully the circle of patience remained unbroken during our winter nights' recreation that holiday season. The mental stimulation benefitted Mother, and she played better each night.

As Christmas day approached, Mother and I finished breakfast at the oval dining room table, which was permanently set with ruffled eyelet place mats. Talking about food for the big day she asked, "Can we have the same thing for Christmas Eve that we have on Christmas day?" My once-fastidious mother wore that same stained sweater again.

Disapproving of leftovers for Christmas dinner, I nixed the idea.

Mother, agitated: "Well, you have those greens to cook. Miz Alice brought them just for you. You need to cook them soon. When are you going to fix them?"

"I'll cook the greens for one of our Christmas meals," I suggested as I began to make a list for grocery shopping.

"I'm NOT serving greens on Christmas!" Leftovers, yes; greens, not so much. Verboten like wearing white after Labor Day.

Mother had been known far and wide for her cooking. She was queen of the kitchen and collector of recipes. She had a drawer full of napkin rings, most of which she had made in her ceramic period. Mother out-Martha'ed Martha Stewart long before that empire existed. However, this year Mother admitted being stressed by days of shopping and cooking for Christmas dinner. I found, in spite of her efforts, only a few things for us to eat. I assumed, that at eighty-five, she was tired from a lifetime of being the lauded cook. It eluded me that tangles in her brain thwarted her ability to organize a meal.

I longed for the Christmas of my youth. Our house highlighted a manger scene on the dining room buffet. The crèche was surrounded by pointy holly leaves maybe less comfortable for baby Jesus than the rank straw in his Last Chance Barn. In those days Mother paraded out all her cooking talents and feats of decoration. A fresh coconut cake was the *piece de resistance*. Daddy cracked the hard brown coconut shell with his hammer, and Mother whipped the sugar-whitened icing in a stovetop stacking of a pan within a pan of boiling water. She did not stop there: she made fudge coated with melted margarine, divinity with and without nuts, and eggnog, thick with egg whites, *sans* alcohol. As Daddy always admonished, "We don't allow any al-ke-hall in this house."

Lately we'd grown accustomed to Sam's Club frozen entrees and no longer expected Mother's kitchen to be warm with the yeasty smell of homemade rolls. But even by those adjusted expectations, Christmas dinner looked paltry, more like Daddy's boyhood holidays. Every year Daddy told us about being a kid in Mississippi: he and his twelve sisters and brothers lucky to get an orange for Christmas. And to make up for his early deprivation, he indulged "his girls," his wife and three daughters. He took us daughters shopping with him for Mother's present. At a neighborhood dress shop, we looked at church clothes, blouses, skirts and fluffy robes.

"What do you think she'd want?" he asked, his insatiable desire to please her especially eager when it came to gifts. "She likes this color, doesn't she?"

Then he had our choices gift-wrapped. The ultimate extravagance.

But this stranger masquerading as my Mother said she was never going to give Christmas presents again. She was definitely missing the joy of the season. I wished Daddy were around to cheer her up and help me understand how to deal with her.

I longed for the Mother who sheltered rather than condemned, the Mother who once made Christmas magic by telling me, "We have a special phone direct to Santa Claus. A secret telephone that calls right up to the North Pole." I believed the magical phone was hidden somewhere in the back reaches of Daddy's business, not as far in the rear as the "colored" bathroom and water fountain, but behind the muffler and air conditioner installation equipment in his automotive garage, where uniformed men were half hidden under hoods of cars and everything reeked of viscous motor oil and gasoline. There were no doubts from me as Mother continued, "I talked to Santa today about that Betsy McCall doll you want him to bring you. Santa was sorry to tell me this, but his elves weren't able to make that for you. Have you seen the Madam Alexander doll? She has the prettiest dress. I can call Santa back and see if the elves can make that." My list, naturally, was long enough to accommodate any elf outages.

Unlike the flimsy artificial tree sitting on an end table in Mother's suburban living room, Christmases past had lights bubbling and blinking on a real tree, redolent with the smell of fresh pine. Underneath the Christmas tree a plethora of presents ensconced in Frosty the Snowman paper tempted our youthful curiosity. We opened nothing early, being children who obeyed. Along with the pink frozen salad, the green bean casserole and the coconut cake, those gifts and other inscrutables went into the trunk of our car and headed to Mississippi for our family holiday traditions. In fact Mother had told Santa, on that private phone to his workshop, that we would be in Mississippi and Santa knew to fulfill our grandest dreams there.

Often it was dusk as our family car moved onto the two-lane highway south to spend Christmas with grandparents, aunts, uncles and cousins. In the back seat we sisters imagined that the farm animals in the barns we passed were celebrating our Savior's birth, gentle like the night of no room at the inn. Along the bumpy roads colored lights led us to the promised land of fire works exploding in the black, country night and lovingly wrapped presents. All that remained to complete our delirious desires was to hang our stockings. My sister Bev and I slept on the scratchy foldout couch in our grandparents' living room, tossing through a sleepless night, wondering what time the grandfather clock's one bell on the half-hour announced. Never once did it occur to me to get up and see what Santa had left under the tree, right beside the sofa where we slept.

We got pogo sticks one Christmas. It was not until adulthood that I heard about Santa's frivolity that night. After eating the cookies, drinking the milk and leaving a thank you note in handwriting strangely like Daddy's, Santa unloaded the loot. In this incarnation as Santa, Mother decided to strut her stuff on the pogo stick. Asleep, we never heard Mother hit the floor giggling, never heard Daddy and the other grown-ups laugh in unaccustomed silliness.

But by 2007 Mother's line to Santa had been disconnected, and her falls were disturbing rather than humorous. Mother had learned to be surreptitious, much like those surprises and regrets delivered in a phone call from the North Pole. Wary of what was obscured in the shadows, I preferred to avoid the whole dilemma and preserve the memory of my compassionate Mother.

I sought to revive Mother's spirit with familiarity. Her church had a Christmas Eve service. I looked forward to this ceremony though to Mother I was now a disappointment as a non-churchgoing adult, especially after being thoroughly entrenched in Southern Baptist life growing up. I started making plans for Mother, Søren and me to go to the Christmas Eve candlelight service.

Mother disagreed. "No, I'm not going. I don't like that young preacher and I can't hear him." Church had always been her epicenter. Mother, a Sunday school teacher, a summer church camp counselor and church scrapbook archivist, loved the Lord. In my youth we even went to church to "pray in" the New Year, on our knees at midnight when others were making champagne toasts and kissing. I did not miss the champagne, being from a pious home that scorned alcohol, but kissing eventually filled my girlhood dreams. In light of such past religious devotion, the Christmas Eve service was *de rigueur*.

Mother put the remaining cups into the dishwasher. "I really don't go to church much any more."

"Is it the driving?"

"No, I can drive just fine. Besides, my friends call and offer to take me. But they're boring." She dropped in the detergent and slammed the dishwasher shut.

What had happened? Had Mother lost her faith? Gotten into a fight with some of her church friends? If only I had known the emotional symptoms of Alzheimer's disease: anxiety, social withdrawal, distrust. The person is unable to join in conversations but is aware of the mental changes and tries to hide the disabilities. Instead, I thought going to church would assuage her fussiness.

I guilted her into going to the candlelight service. A Christmas tree of red poinsettias filled the foyer of the church. In the unlit sanctuary we sang "Silent Night," then each worshipper lit the candle of the next person in the church pew. Illumination blessed the congregation, dispersing the darkness. Sharing a small flame enlightened each of us. The promise of radiance penetrated the dimness of my despondency about Mother. When Mother greeted her friends with good cheer, I considered myself the Christmas angel, lighting her gloom.

No amount of denial could hide the fact that Mother had declined significantly. Both of my sisters, Bev and Judy, had been in Memphis the previous summer. We continually commiserated about Mother's recent intractability, but neither had been overly concerned about her. She had always been stubborn. After all, aging was normal, absentmindedness expected. And to call on Jung again, if we admitted Mother's problems, it would leave us "orphaned and isolated," on the edge of umbra.

After Søren went back to Cincinnati, Mother lost a set of keys. It became the end of the world, the Confederacy losing the War Between the States, and a spark in her brain that burned a hole and set her anxiety aflame.

"I had my neighbor's front door key on there. What will they think?" she bemoaned as she frantically stuck her age-spotted hands behind peach and white sofa cushions and opened kitchen drawers. "What if somebody finds the keys and breaks into Marie's condo?"

I followed behind her, lifting chair cushions and reaching into the pockets of her long brown coat hanging in the living room closet. "They're around here somewhere."

"This is awful."

"Let's think about this. When did you have them last?" If I hadn't been at Mother's, I would have opened a beer.

She pointed. "I always put them right on that hook by the back door."

"What about these keys?" I asked grabbing a set hanging on the hook, thinking my work accomplished. "These have a house key and a car key."

"That's not the set with Marie's condo key on it!" Mother opened a kitchen cabinet. Then another.

"We'll just get copies of your keys made. I'm sure Marie's daughter has other keys for her condo."

"What could've happened to them?" She hurried back to her den and I heard more drawers opening. Closing.

"Let's just go get another set made. Isn't there a hardware store near your bank?"

"We're not leaving. I know those keys are around here somewhere." The vertical wrinkles between her deep-set blue eyes intensified, leaving crevices of worry. She rubbed herself unconsciously. "Marie's key was on that key ring."

"People lose their keys all the time. It's not a big deal." At last I got her to agree to have another set made, but she would not consider getting them from the hardware store in her neighborhood.

"We'll go over to Highland. I know those people who have a locksmith shop there."

"That's a long drive for just a couple of keys, and we don't really need a locksmith," I noted, though admitting to myself we had nothing but time.

"No! We're going to Highland. They know your dad had a business on Highland. I know them. We're going where they know me."

We gathered our winter coats, and I took the remaining set of keys out to the garage. I always drove in Memphis. It was one of the few responsibilities Mother would allow her daughters, and we all suspected she did not want us to see her behind the wheel, since we had begun to question her driving. Arriving at the locksmith,

Mother went in and asked for the owner. I stood nearby fidgeting with the keys in my coat pocket to distract myself from Mother's performance. The owner was away for Christmas vacation.

"We just need a few keys made," I interjected, stepping forward.

"I can take care of this!" Mother eyeballed me with withering skills resurrected to put me in my place. She lost not a beat, needing to know when the owner was returning. Then she turned on her Southern charm, someone playing scales, each note practiced to perfection. "My husband owned the Esso service station down the street on Highland. For thirty-four years. Something happened to a set of my keys."

I laid down her key ring. The woman at the counter explained that it would cost $25 to have the car key copied.

Mother was irate. "Well, I don't need another car key. I'm going to find that other key ring." Again she asked when the owner was coming back.

All of Highland must have heard me sigh. "Well, let's just get a house key made, to be on the safe side." Later, researching Alzheimer's, I learned that normally folks adjusted to the inconvenience of misplaced keys, but with dementia daily problems seemed insurmountable.

No doubt the poor woman at the counter had never worked any harder for a couple of dollars, though she didn't grimace during Mother's repetitions. Perhaps later at home when the woman retold of her day at work in one long breath she said, "This elderly woman, bless her heart, was really upset about losing her keys."

Mother, bless her heart, was still fretting about the lost keys when we finally got back to the suburbs as the gray day gave up the last rays of thin light.

Being in Memphis darkened my perspective. I hid in the guest bedroom with contraband wine in a coffee cup, wondering how I would dispose of the empty bottle. Though "alkeehall" was always a demon to my parents, Mother had become even more obsessed about it. I feared the alcohol-police finding the evidence and sentencing me to a life of sobriety living with Mother. Originally the constitution protected against cruel and unusual punishment, but times had changed, and I might be doomed.

One evening I decided to cook for myself. I wanted to update my southern roots and use Mother's cast-iron skillet for a grilled pimento cheese sandwich. That skillet was the longtime site of red-eye gravy for breakfast, fried chicken and creamed corn for supper. Without Velveeta it was not my mother's pimento cheese. Still I spread the cheddar and Gouda pimento cheese on dense wheat bread and pulled the skillet from the lower cabinet. Through half of the skillet was a crack wide enough to let in light. How hot did the skillet get to burst like that? I had always assumed an iron skillet could take very high heat, but this cracked skillet had sat forgotten on an electric burner turned onto high, and I realized the shortcomings of a metal I had thought almost indestructible. The companion spatula, handle melted away, laid in the drawer. I stood in Mother's personal space and cried.

Chapter 4

TEAM LOU

"Memory is a complicated thing, a relative to truth, but not its twin."

Barbara Kingsolver

Memphis, Christmas 2007

Mother managed to keep it together for short periods of time. On her better days, as one Memphis friend explained, she appeared "really sharp mentally." She could pay her bills. She still wrote lovely thank you notes in a graceful, slanting script. She spent hours talking on the phone. Her friends in the condominium community appreciated how she often shared food with them. In summer she put on her tan Bermuda shorts and, baring her legs, skin protruding with knotty veins, sat beside the condominium swimming pool with her neighbors. She had collected the sympathetic attention of good neighbors, relatives, and church friends.

Foremost among Mother's affectionate fan club was Alex. When we were in high school, Mother and Daddy extended a truly generous open house policy for our teen-age friends, who as adults had stayed in touch with Mother and Daddy. Alex* in

* Alex is not his real name, though he is a real person. I renamed him in homage to "Summons to Memphis" by Peter Taylor: one of my favorite books, set, where else, but in Memphis. In "Summons to Memphis" the narrator, who moved away from Memphis, had a best friend from high

particular loved my openhearted parents, and Alex's wife Sandra would drop food off for Mother, hanging bags of homemade meals on the back gate. Consequently, Mother called on Alex quite often for assistance. On Sunday afternoon, braving the raw weather in Memphis, I visited Alex and Sandra. I needed Memphis partners to acknowledge what I saw as a disturbing reality, something along the lines of boll weevils decimating the cotton crops.

(Take heart. Boll weevils, those microscopic pests, were eradicated in the 1950s. Wiped out by DDT, before DDT was banned because of the exposure in "Silent Spring" and the environmental movement. But that's a bead for another rosary, a deadly solution, and pentimento landscapes.)

"Oh, Alex, you did such an incredible job on this house," I admired. He had been contractor, carpenter and craftsman in restoring their lovely 1920s home where I sat in their living room.

"I know," Sandra agreed. "He's such an artist."

As we talked, I told them about a few incidents with Mother, and I started to cry. "I'm just so concerned about her. I don't know what to do." Sucking in short breaths between tears, I tried to explain that my sisters and I wanted to help Mother. I cried some more. "I'm sorry, I didn't know I was so upset."

"Of course you are, she's your mama," Sandra acknowledged.

"We really want her to move near one of us so we can take care of her."

---

school, who remained good friends with the narrator's parents. This best friend, Alex, communicated with the parents and the narrator, listening compassionately, and went to the Memphis airport when the narrator returned for a visit. This is also the true story of my so-called Alex. He respected my parents and always met me at the airport, no matter how late my flight. Alex was like the son my mother never had. Every family should be so lucky to have a caring and dependable Alex in their life.

"Mama Walls," that's what Alex called Mother, "doesn't want to move, and she doesn't want to lose her independence."

My voice, resorting to encoded Southern cadences, trembled. "But she's already lost her independence. She can't drive at night and she misses out on most conversations." I wanted Alex and Sandra to be our allies in getting Mother resituated. "I'm afraid something's going to happen to her. We want to prevent any disasters."

Alex and Sandra sat in their beautifully upholstered chairs, watching me cry. I realized they were a part of Team Lou, the bless-her-heart chorus, along with the aunts, cousins and neighbors who were slightly removed from the depth of the problem.

Heading back to Mother's I pulled the car over on a quiet street. The seemingly empty, large brick houses sat back on the brown front yards, the leafless tree branches unmoving in the cold air. From that desolation I called Aunt Donna Lynn.

She said to me, "Were you surprised by how much your mother's gone down hill this year? I've been so worried about her."

I thanked her for telling me, saying it was hard to evaluate what was happening. The vista outside Mother's Buick was flat and bare; I was far away from the distinct white crowns of the mountain ranges in my beloved state of Washington. I told Aunt Donna Lynn we wanted Mother to move near one of us so that we could take care of her, but she warned me, "Lou would fight that. She doesn't wanna move." Never once in these Memphis discussions was the possibility of Alzheimer's mentioned.

Team Lou tended to agree with Mother's wishes. What did they think we were going to do, leave our jobs, homes and families and move to Memphis to take care of her? Our best option was moving her near one of us. I was grateful when one of my aunts, dressed in a red sweater happy with snowmen, admitted to me, "I can see your side, but I can see her side, too."

Each daughter had talked to Mother about assisted living, sent her literature about facilities in our hometowns and offered to move her near us. Søren cracked up when I told him about the letter and pamphlets I had sent, suggesting that it was time for her to move, proposing she look at moving as an adventure. He found it hysterical I thought the idea of adventure would persuade her. (Out of the mouths of babes.)

Mother had a standard response to our pleas for her to move: "The Lord's going to take me in my sleep at home." This was Mother's version of "it's a beeeuuuutiful day." Calling on the Lord to take her in her sleep at home was not only a signal to end that particular conversation, but never to begin it again. After all, who could argue with divine intervention? Rationally we suggested, just in case, she might need an alternative plan.

But even Mother couldn't let go of the subject. She pulled it out again, like a Crisco-stained 3X5 recipe card. "I won't have to move. The Lord's going to take me in my sleep at home."

"How's that working for your friends?" Bev had once countered.

Not wanting to talk about the deaths of so many who had been precious to her, Mother feigned, putting the familiar card back in the reliable recipe box. "Only kidding."

Late one afternoon I sat on a tall stool facing Mother in her compact kitchen. Mother and I were both worn out from our hostilities, and asking Mother questions about her youth became a welcome reprieve from our battles. Her long-term memory remained in tact as her short-term memory faltered. As John Updike wrote, "In memory's telephoto lens, far objects are magnified." Her lanky frame had the fluidity of a choir robe while she made supper. I opened a small leather notebook, placing it on the white cabinet top where Mother both ate and talked on the telephone. Clutter collected around the white phone. I was scribbling notes onto the rice paper in my little notebook, needing to write all this down before it was too late. There were many in Mother's history, relatives of mine, also, who were only names on a chart to me, landmarks, peripheral shadows on the topography of her life.

I prodded Mother. "Remember how Papa Vinson called Judy and Bev and me 'girl' and never by our names? And he called Daddy, 'Walls'?" I had often wondered what was buried beneath Papa Vinson's reticence, looking for what motivated him to take a leadership role in his community as an adult.

"That's how people talked. Besides, Papa Vinson grew up hard." Mother explained returning to a family refrain. "His father died when Papa was just a boy." Mother took some creamed corn out of the refrigerator and poured it in a pan. "Papa Vinson's daddy died before Aunt Willie was born."

"So Aunt Willie was Papa Vinson's younger sister? Is that why you were named after her?" Papa Vinson's newly born, fatherless baby sister was named Willie Mae, and my mother, decades later, was brought into this world as Willie Lou Vinson. In the mold of most double-name holders, as an adult she preferred only one name, dropped Willie and was called Lou. There were very few people still alive who were allowed the intimacy of addressing her as Willie Lou.

"Papa and Aunt Willie were close. But that was later. After his father died, when Papa was a boy and Aunt Willie was a baby, they moved in with Ma's parents, the Robbins family. Ma is what we called Papa Vinson's mother," she continued. "Papa Vinson was one of a passel of boys and all of them were his uncles, his granddaddy's sons. He was somewhere in the middle. When Ma remarried, Papa Vinson didn't go to live with Ma and his stepfather. He stayed in the house with his uncles and grandparents. Ma's new husband wasn't any good and we didn't like him."

"What did Ma's new husband do?"

"Oh, I don't know. Not much. He was a farmer like everybody else."

"What was Ma like?" I asked, adding names to my family tree.

"Well, she wasn't talkative or affectionate," Mother shrugged. It seemed to me that when it came to Papa Vinson, the apple didn't fall far from that tree. Mother mused, finally turning down the heat on the corn, which was boiling furiously, "Do you remember how before he died Papa would ask over and over to go out and see the boys in the yard? He was remembering his uncles when they were kids together." That boyhood time for Papa Vinson was etched deeply like dry rows in a late summer garden; one of his last wishes was once more to join in their company, romping in Mississippi fields, never alone even when death grazed beside those rough country roads.

I continued. "You had a lot of family living with you when you were young."

"I guess so. There was Granny Susie, Mama Mat's mother. I loved Granny and I was her favorite. She was so sweet. She had a hard life too. She died when I was about seven or eight years old. Ma Robbins moved in when I was teaching at Boyle." With the passage of time Ma Robbins had become a widow for the second time. She moved in with Papa Vinson and Mama Mat and died in their home in Ellistown.

Hearing Mother's fond memories about the relatives who lived with them, I wished she could transfer that communal spirit into moving close to her daughters. But I didn't want to start another altercation, so I stayed with the questions about the past. "I remember that Aunt Willie and her daughter Florence lived with you after Aunt Willie's husband died of diabetes. Weren't Florence and Aint E about the same age?"

"They graduated from high school the same year."

"Where were you living?" I was tracking an atlas of Mother's life, even as the maps in her brain became tattered with detours and dead ends, calling forth her early connections to secure her with me in the present.

"We had moved back to Ellistown. Papa had gotten a different store. So Elois and Florence drove back to Sherman, where we used to live, to finish high school."

"Aint E had a car? Wow."

"Just a little roadster. What average people had," Mother explained to defer my notion of opulence. "A Chevy or a Ford. Do you want some iced tea?" Mother got glasses from the overhead cabinet. "Elois was Papa's favorite, though. If anybody in the family wanted anything, even Mama Mat, we would get Elois to ask Papa."

"Papa Vinson had a soft spot for Aint E. How sweet. Did Papa get mad at you and not at her?" I questioned, shaking my head "no" as Mother reached for the plastic tea pitcher, stained by years of tannins. "Water's fine. Do you want any help?"

"Here, take these plates." And she passed me two gold-rimmed plates decorated with magnolias. "No, Papa didn't get mad." Then she told me a story about Papa Vinson's temperament as we sat down to eat.

MISSISSIPPI PAST

Mother was in college, apparently, and the roads were muddy from rain. Mother and her friend Earline wanted to go somewhere and asked Papa Vinson if they could borrow the car. Papa Vinson said yes, but don't go to Mary Rose's house, the roads are too bad. Off Mother and Earline went to (where else?) Mary Rose's; maybe Mother was driving too fast, or perhaps the rut-slashed roads diverted her, but they ended up stuck in a ditch, mired in red mud. The roads were, indeed, bad. Stalled there, panicked, another car with two men drove up behind them, and Mother winced. It was Papa Vinson in that car. With no conversation, nary a word, Papa Vinson and his friend pushed Mother's car back onto the road and drove away. Mother worried, knowing she was in trouble for disobeying Papa Vinson, and when she got back home she went to her room and hid, ever the brave college student. For days she was upset, but Papa Vinson never mentioned the incident.

Memphis 2007

While Mother and I reminisced, she was relaxed and chatty, the tension in her shoulders and mouth dissipated. On the phone later that night I told Bev, "She may actually like me again."

Cell phones and emails were my salvation during that bitter December in Memphis. Somehow I hitched my laptop onto a neighbor's Wi-Fi and poured my misgivings across cyberspace. Technology was my friend and my lifeline. Tucked away in Mother's guest bedroom, fancy with her best antiques, I was supported by my sisters in my apprehensions about Mother.

Bev emailed: *I've been wondering if she needs to be checked for Alzheimer's or dementia. That anger that is festering all the time and flares up unexpectedly can be a symptom of Alzheimer's. She's paranoid that we're after her money. We definitely need someone coming in regularly to be our eyes and ears and for her, a soothing, helping hand. Mom covers up a lot.*

I think that we don't have much longer to get her on board for moving. I do understand that it must look like the end of life as she knows it, but she'd enjoy being around other people, having someone else's cooking to complain about, getting waited on. I think that she's too isolated, too lonely.

My sisters and I decided to begin a file on our computers to evaluate Mother's changes, a tool that we might need when we talked to doctors. After an intense conversation a sister would admonish, "Put that in the Lou Report!" The Lou Report was a reality check for any refusal on our part to face facts, a reminder for when we looked instead at the beeeutiful day. A useful tool, but I felt disloyal at the same time. Since then I have seen such a list suggested in books for Alzheimer's caregivers as an aid in an overwhelming process: an inventory to keep the rush of events in perspective. The books were right, but those books could not hear Mother's hiss in my conscience about how mean it was to emphasize her imperfections. After all, I forgot things too. What if someone made this kind of catalogue about me?

I emailed my sisters: *Do you think we're each a little bit afraid of Mother? Otherwise we would swoop in, move her and get on with our lives. I've thought several times on this visit that I need to see a therapist when I get home. This is serious business, switching life-long roles. You should've heard Søren's blessing to the God of mercy: forgive us our vanity, our pride, our idiocy, our impatience, our lack of love. Afterwards I said, wow, you nailed me on all counts. Somehow it wasn't judgmental, but an honest airing of our flaws.*

My visit was drawing to an end and throughout the two weeks with Mother I had heard her recite the same complaints and worries many times over. Like that old car in college, Mother was stuck in a quagmire about Aint E's death. No matter how many questions I asked about Mother's youth, she got the conversation back to Aint E's funeral. It had taken place on a windy November morning in Mississippi only a month prior. My sisters and I admitted to Mother and our selves that Mother would never move as long as Elois was alive. But Elois had died, and with that Mother's last excuse. Did Mother also realize she had lost her last rationale for staying in Memphis?

When Aint E was dying, Mother called me several times a day. I asked her what Aint E was like as a sister. Mother replied that as a girl Elois could do five or six cartwheels across their front yard. I could see Aint E, light and carefree, twirling barefoot across a barren space in northern Mississippi. "And I couldn't even do one," Mother marveled, the little sister still admiring the talents of her big sis. During Aint E's end days as my cousins sat beside her bed, I envisioned her cartwheeling into her Baptist Heaven, leaving behind the crippling fog of Parkinson's, gleeful to be approaching the Light of her Creator. Both Mother and I missed Elois; however Mother had lost not only a dear sister but also a treasured purpose. Thus, the stress of grief most likely increased Mother's troubling symptoms.

When I returned to Seattle after Christmas I wrote Mother a card saying I was sorry for our disagreements. I never said I was wrong or she was impossible, just that I wished we had not had such a tough time. I wanted to make everything better. What daughter doesn't?

An email from Bev later in January: *Mother is basically dismissing us, giving back her hearing aid, and going back into hibernation.*

She also told Judy that she's not at a point that she needs anyone coming in to drive her or check on her. "I don't need to be paying for that."

I emailed my sisters: *I hope Daddy, however the afterlife works, understands that we're doing the best we can for Mother. He, of all people, must have scars from her stubbornness.*

I remember during the last decade of his life Daddy would say, "life's too short" in answer to every question. He thought life was too short to spend being unhappy and encouraged moving on. I don't recall what caused him to offer that insight, but later I came to think he felt there was not enough time for all he loved and enjoyed. If only Mother understood that: life is too short to be lonely, to fight, to resist inevitable change. However, whatever is happening in her brain has confused her on a level that we can't negotiate. I only hope her prayers are strong enough to protect her; because it doesn't seem like she's going to let us help her.

Chapter 5

THE SCIENCE OF YOUR BRAIN ON ALZHEIMER'S

"While I've always wanted to get people's stories, I also like to know what's going on in the brain, and how this wonderful two or three pounds of stuff in the head is able to underlie our imagination, underlie our soul and our individuality."

Dr. Oliver Sacks, neurologist

A BRIEF TOUR OF THE BRAIN

As the decay of Alzheimer's disease spreads, the facilities of the brain are impaired and even destroyed. The brain directs it all: memory, passion, bodily functions, walking, and the complete list of operating in this physical world. With Alzheimer's disease the director has lost power and the movie is fading from the big screen.

THE LIMBIC SYSTEM

The present medical consensus is that Alzheimer's disease (AD) begins in the hippocampus, where new memories are made.[1,2] The hippocampus is buried deep inside the cranium, in the innermost fold of the temporal lobe, in the limbic part of the brain. The limbic system, known as the ancient or reptilian brain, is the emotional site. Here, in the most basic of assemblage, feelings and memory connect.[3,4] The strongest arousals, the person, the book, the experience that made the big splashes in this emotional pool, those swim on as memories. The hippocampus has the job of transferring such incoming information into retention. Without this ability to make new memories, there is no living in the present. Thoughts and images evaporate, leaving only the past. Learning is lost. (And oh what a loss!) Without the power to make new memories, there are daily questions like "where is my purse," "what was it we did this morning," or, even worse, a panic about the cause of a burning skillet. Without the ability to put thoughts into long-term memory, repetitive questions may arise. Mother, her hippocampus damaged, would ask the same question over and over, a true test to the patience of her daughters and grandchildren.

The hippocampus turns sensory information, thoughts, impressions, emotional responses and even scents into long-term memory.[5] In fact, the hippocampus interprets information and organizes it into long-term retrieval systems by cross-association and contextualizing.[6] Would that mean the hippocampus is our Google and it becomes a weakened search engine as the brain deteriorates? If only there was IT help for the hippocampus.

Spatial recognition may originate from the hippocampus, making it the navigational center of the brain for complex and visual discrimination.[7] In studying taxi drivers in 2000 in London, who found their way without GPS, but rather by using visual sightings and the experience of finding new routes and shortcuts, scientists discovered that those cab drivers had larger hippocampi than other people.[8] This may provide another explanation about AD patients getting lost. If the cognitive map in their hippocampus is damaged, they might no longer have the internal GPS to find their way home.

Alzheimer's, the clandestine disease, takes root in the hippocampus, clogging this essential center, evaporating sensations. If a person can't know what just happened, it becomes difficult to assess time and place. Consequently, on cognitive tests to screen for dementia, patients are asked simple questions about where and when. The wrong answers indicate deterioration in the hippocampus. With these losses, the cascade of uncertainty escalates.

Also a part of the limbic system is the amygdala, which regulates basic feelings like fear, anger, and craving.[9] Motivation, a guiding force of behavior, takes shape here. In the amygdala social behavior is modified into appropriate responses.[10] With this center disturbed, the unexplained behavior starts: the outbursts, the where-did-that-come-from fury, and the obsessive anxiety. Much to the chagrin of family, strangers are criticized, and an unexplained moment spirals into embarrassment. Newer studies are suggesting amygdala disruption in early AD may play a role in patients' depression and anxiety.[11]

The brain stem, also found in the limbic region, is often affected early in Alzheimer's. Sleep patterns are disrupted;[12] another torturous change for the patient. Here is a person, extremely anxious about mental changes, awake in the dark; now add sleep deprivation to the equation. Cognitive function is disturbed for a healthy person from this exhausted state; this would be compounded for a person with dementia. The person, once bright with accomplishments, is already becoming a flickering candle. Sundowning syndrome, restlessness and confusion manifested as sunset brings on shadows, starts.[13] Late in AD, the functions of the brain stem change such vital processes as breathing, blood pressure, and heart rate.[14] This or some other complication, perhaps pneumonia or the inability to swallow, may cause death.

THE FRONTAL LOBES

The frontal lobes are the home of purposeful behavior and complex reasoning such as making plans, evaluations, considering threats, and long periods of concentration.[15] For both the young and AD patients, complex problem solving is not fully supported, nor is planning for the future. With deterioration in the frontal lobes logic is compromised;[16] decisions lack fundamental reasoning, and complicated activities become giant obstacles. In AD skills like balancing a checkbook or getting a dead battery fixed are thwarted. When the frontal lobes are damaged by the disease, there is likely little or no reasoning with someone with AD. These patients aren't being willful; their brain has lost processing skills. We kept saying about Mother, "It's like we can't reason with her." Yet we continued to try to reason with her, as a way to get her to change her mind.

When frontal and amygdala problems combine, there is a loss of inhibition, the mortifying moments of swearing, saying mean things loudly in the doctor's reception area, and toward the end undressing in public. Mother would proclaim shrilly, much to her daughters' dismay, "That woman is so fat!" or "That's an ugly dress she's wearing!" We wanted a t-shirt or a card with an apology, please excuse our mother, she has Alzheimer's. If she had a cane, people would sympathize with her slow gait. Physical illnesses are visible and gleam sympathy. AD symptoms like rudeness, on the other hand, can be misunderstood, even by family.

THE PARIETALS

The parietals are the site of motor and sensory skills, of control and awareness of the body, of orienting ourselves to the space and the things around us.[17] Bumping into things might be a result of parietal damage. When this rich brain soil, which grows words into thoughts, is engulfed by mental kudzu, wandering, getting lost at home, and mixing up objects become prominent. Mother would walk into a room, muttering, "What am I doing here? Where am I going?" While we've all done that, the ability to link ideas and information is another casualty. Sensory input about temperature, touch, pain, and pressure is recognized and interpreted in this brain region.[16] A plethora of burns, bruises, and other injuries may be an indicator at this stage of the AD brain sweep.

When AD affects parietal lobes, it challenges the internal representations of personal navigation.[17] This progress in the disease can result in a lack of coordination, not being able to interpret cracks in the sidewalk, or not distinguishing distances. Another symptom easy to misinterpret. When my aunt was describing Mother's decline, she said, "The way she walks." And her neighbors said of Mother, "She's so healthy, except that she falls a lot." I noticed the way she shuffled, but we excused theses symptoms because she had osteoporosis. Besides, haven't we all seen the elderly hobbling around with their canes, tripping over a curb? We automatically think aging and don't consider Alzheimer's disease as the cause. However, studies have found that "motion blindness" may explain the disorientation of AD patients.[18]

Deterioration in the Medial Superior Temporal area (MST) may cause "motion blindness" and spatial problems. Motion detection arises in the MST, where background motion is distinguished from personal movement.[19] Because of changes in this part of the brain, motion becomes invisible to AD patients; they do not see movement, they see only a series of stills, a scrapbook rather than a video. When this motion interpreter in the brain goes down, the person cannot process visual information about movement, depth or color,[20] which influences the patient's own movement, walking, and particularly disorientation. The MST, rather than memory loss, may be another cause of wandering and getting lost. With deterioration in the MST, other hazards persist. The patient may not be able to detect the movement of others. Can she actually see that car moving? Does he recognize that the door is closing? Understanding this part of the disease underscores any concern about driving a car, even for someone exhibiting early symptoms of AD. Motion blindness may be another explanation for why Mother quit watching television, once her household background hum, or why she tripped fell so often. We insisted on taking Mother to get new glasses. Surely that was her problem, not some little known area of her parietals. It must be her eyes rather than brain issues.

TEMPORAL LOBES

The temporal lobes could be likened to computer memory: this is the place of information storage and its recovery, home of long-term memory, language, and understanding speech.[21] Early AD in this section presents with aphasia, difficulty with words and with naming things.[22] (Instead of "over draft" Mother said "over checked.") Concepts become more difficult to articulate. Later damage in the temporals is expressed in auditory and visual hallucinations.[23]

BDNF AND NEUROGENESIS

For healthy brains, there's good news about cerebral functioning. For decades scientists believed the brain was fixed, limited to the neurons that shaped the brain at birth and during the explosive growth of childhood. It was believed that neurons could not regenerate, and therefore, humans were stuck with an unchanging number of neurons, which decreased with age and illness, particularly with brain-degenerative diseases. By 2002 The Journal of Neuroscience published an article stating, "A milestone is marked in our understanding of the brain with the recent acceptance, contrary to early dogma, that the adult nervous system can generate new neurons." Now neurogenesis, the brain's ability to grow and develop neurons throughout adulthood, is known to be an important mechanism enabling humans to learn and adapt.[24] The article further qualifies that two areas of the brain can generate new neurons: the hippocampus and the subventricular zone.[21] Hallelujah! Humans are not stuck with an immutable brain! Our brains are malleable, moldable, like clay; this ability of the adult brain to grow neurons and new neuronal pathways is known as neuroplasticity.[24] What potential our brains have! Our brains can adapt to our needs, can reorganize synaptic connections from new information, and can replace lost neurons.

DNA and neural stem cells, not surprisingly, influence neurogenesis. Supporting roles are performed by neurotrophins, a family of proteins or chemicals that stimulate neurogenesis. Think of Brain-Derived Neurotrophic Factor (BDNF) as the starring neurotrophin for creating neurons.* Dr. John Ratey of Harvard, in his book "SPARK: The Revolutionary New Science of Exercise and the Brain," described BDNF as fertilizer for this neuronal growth.[25] BDNF binds to receptors in the synapses between neurons, promoting protective pathways for neuron growth and survival. It is a crucial link between thought, emotions and movement. BDNF's sites of activity include the hippocampus, the cortex and other brain

* Not to complicate an already complex subject, but BDNF is also a gene as well as a protein; however, this book will be considering only the workings of the BDNF protein

areas vital to learning, memory and higher thinking.[26,27] As might be expected, studies have shown decreased BDNF in Alzheimer's patients, as well as lower BDNF in a variety of neurological conditions including Parkinson's Disease.

Everything I read has confirmed that we are in the beginning of the process of understanding the brain. New technologies continue to open windows for seeing into brain functioning, though any knowledge can be usurped by the next discovery. In the words of astrophysicist Neil deGrasse Tyson, "Exactly how the human brain operates remains one of the biggest unsolved mysteries, and it seems the more we probe its secrets, the more surprises we find."[28]

Chapter 6

Y'ALL WAITED TOO LATE

"Her children wouldn't have understood, she didn't herself, how even peripheral people had taken up the space in her life that they had once occupied."
Stanley Elkin, Mrs. Ted Bliss

Memphis, April 2008

Spring in magnolia-shaded Memphis, and Mother and I walked around the graceful grounds of her condominium village. Mother seemed a little wobbly, and I gently took her arm. She was still dressed in the peach shirt and navy blue slacks that she'd worn to the doctor's office that morning. Her cheeks, round like Howdy-Doody's, that cheerful puppet from childhood television, were rosy with excitement.

She said, "See that hosta, I gave it to Carol. Isn't it pretty?" The leaf mimed a bold hue of blue, pretty like the cloudless sky. I could picture Mother, digging in her flowerbeds with her elegant hands, separating out the hosta plants, shaking the soil from the roots. "Look at that white azalea. Oh! Hi boy!" Mother leaned down to pet the tethered basset hound, his jowls and stomach skimming the ground. "He belongs to Carol. I wonder if she's home. Let's knock on her door."

Carol wasn't home and we continued down the concrete walkway, admiring the irises. A plaster bust of Elvis, his shirt collar brushing his gorgeous cheekbones, held center stage among the flowers. "Now, what did we do today?" Mother inquired.

"We went to get you a bone density test."

"We did?"

I was in Memphis to check on Mother, to reconcile after the debacle of the previous Christmas, and in hopes of rebuilding trust with a peaceful visit. When I told Soren this, he kidded, "I'd pay money to see you not have an argument with her for three days." But I was on a mission, and none of her criticisms about me, my sisters, or other relatives, none of her barbs, not even her convoluted driving directions hooked my latent teen-aged rebellion.

Remembering what upset her in December, I ate everything on my plate. I even ate the pink frozen salad, individually formed into muffin baking cups, colored by the red dye of canned maraschino cherries, waiting in her freezer (for who knows how long) to complement any meal. We went to doctors' appointments, though they didn't stick in her memory. It was all very light, and her lapses reminded me of a happy drunk: my teetotaler mom, *sans* booze as always, acting slightly tipsy and on a lark. To her credit she made jokes, named plants, and told stories. As I reassured Bev, "We had fun."

After my visit with Mother at Christmas, we had begun in earnest our sisterly movement to rescue Mother. More visits, making trips for doctor's visits, more phone calls, more involved. One of us went to Memphis at least every other month. Judy was the most frequent visitor, buckling up her seat belt and driving across the elongated state of Tennessee. Mother seemed to have more minor health issues. Prescriptions were needed, and we were determined to convince her to see things our way. We also attempted to manage her from our homes, not always successfully.

Team Lou in Memphis not withstanding, we daughters were pressing for change. We sincerely wanted to look after her in these, the last years of her life. Having watched the outside care necessary for several of our aunts in assisted living, and even discounting the basic need for tangible family love, we did not feel that planting her in an assisted living facility in Memphis with her daughters spread across the country would be the best choice. In telling my cousin Brock about this, he had no doubt: "Y'all waited too late. You'll never get her to move now." Though discouraged, I refused to believe that was true. It could always be a beeeauuuuuutiful day in my mind.

Promises were made and deadlines set, later ignored. We picked up our letter writing to encourage Mother in our direction, expressing great tenderness, making suggestions about in-home care, confessing the entire crazy quilt of feelings. We begged Mother not to be angry and implored Daddy as our support. Nothing like a dead dad to bolster our side. These were magnificent, pleading letters that would have been better sent at least five years earlier, before the disturbances. Mother would say she got our letters, but she would never discuss them with us. It did not deter us from writing, nor did we ever consider that she was unable to perceive the words, the paragraphs, or the meaning. The terrain of her brain, overgrown with tau and plaque, was concealed from us. In that way my cousin Brock was right, we had waited too late.

When I stopped in Memphis that spring pink with azaleas, I was on my way to New Orleans for Jazzfest, and it tweaked Mother's memory. She told me about her early vacations with Daddy.

VACATIONS PAST

Mother and Daddy flew to New Orleans, an early airplane trip for both of them. Daddy was still trying to impress her. Flying must have been an exquisite exception from long drives they knew so well in hot automobiles; an escape from those car trips with the windows rolled down, the wind a stinging breath as skin stuck to the stiff seats in southern humidity. What a luxurious contrast they found in airline travel. Naturally they dressed up; he in his best Sunday suit and she with gloves. A totally different flying epoch. Mother was pregnant with me. Flying through the upper reaches the plane took a sudden plunge and the custard pie being eaten stuck to the ceiling or smeared on blouses. Yes, there was a dessert course. It was 1946. Stewardesses hurried to clean up the embarrassing mess.

On another trip, when I was about two years old, Daddy took us to Eureka Springs, Arkansas. Mother was very excited about the vacation and anticipated going to a nice motel. She was probably pregnant with Bev at that time. Daddy serviced the black Oldsmobile at his Esso station before the trip. As it turned out, the motel was "out in the country" and not so modern, nothing to compare with Mother's imagination of how posh the accommodations would be. Daddy took the suitcases from the trunk of the black car into a small bungalow. Pine needles from the hovering trees carpeted the path to the screen door. It was not the vacation of her dreams. During the night some forest animal got in the motel room and ran around madly. Mother screamed, trying to protect me, while Daddy went after the intruder. The culprit was much smaller than Mother's fears. But what scared her when I was little had us both chuckling pleasantly as silver-haired adults. I thought about how fears, like unknown animals in the darkness, plagued her now. Life cheated her daily of her reveries, her daughters' demands like noisy invasions, and Daddy no longer around to quiet her scurrying thoughts.

SUMMER 2008

I left Memphis feeling confident. Mother hadn't been paranoid, and I thought we could negotiate our way through future dilemmas. Even with the best of intentions, though, things could turn ugly fast. Mother had no medical diagnosis of mental inabilities, and we were left without legal power or palpable alternatives.

Here were our medical concerns: mental decline, hypothyroid (she had thyroid surgery years ago), and high blood pressure. Mother had a cardiologist downtown, who prescribed her hypertension meds. By the time she drove there, probably got lost, and finally found a parking spot, her systolic blood pressure was over 200. Definitely a bad number. Mother had erased the cardiologist from her calendar, despite phone calls from his office. As for general care, Mother's desired doc couldn't take her as a patient because of some Medicare snafu.

Somehow we talked Mother into seeing a neurologist for her back and leg pains. Our surreptitious agenda was also to get a consultation on her mental health. Judy had the dirty job of taking Mother to that appointment. My youngest sister is practical, hard working, compassionate of elders, and always, a woman of action. That's probably how we all think of her: making Thanksgiving for thirty people, making lists, making things happen. A woman in charge. The Little General moving her troops.

By the time Judy and her husband Buddy got to Memphis, Mother had cancelled the neurologist's appointment. Judy was frank, too frank for Mother's taste, and firewater blazed in Mother's prohibitionist soul. Judy addressed Mother's failing abilities. She expressed worry about the kitchen fires, about the memory loss and Mother's driving. Judy said something like "I just hope you don't have a wreck and kill somebody else." To whatever Judy suggested as a solution, Mother screamed like a furious two-year-old, "You! Can't! Make! Me!"

Judy told both Bev and me about the argument, but Mother didn't. Much of our family history is based on pretend. Pretend the fight didn't happen. Act like you never heard about it. Imagine the Rebels didn't lose the War of the Secession.

Weeks after the blowout with Judy, I called Mother. The first thing she said, making me a speaker of untruth, was "Has Judy called you?" And not in her molasses voice.

"What?" I asked.

"Have you talked to Judy?"

I lied. May I be forgiven, but I said "no" because we were all aware that Mother saw us sisters as "piling on." Southern women know football and can recognize "piling on" when they see it.

In my conversation with Mother the word Alzheimer's came up often. She said, "They're trying to prove I have Alzheimer's."

If only I had agreed, "Yes, you might have Alzheimer's." My responses often came back to wanting to please Mother, as it was essential in our upbringing not to make her ashamed of our behavior. The last time I got spanked, I had stuck my tongue out at Bev, across the church aisles. "That embarrassed your mother," Daddy chided, before taking his belt to the teen-aged me at her insistence. On the phone with Mother, adult-to-adult, the way she said the word Alzheimer's it could only be an affront, the worst thing we could say about her. I didn't want to stop the openness between us by embarrassing her with a verdict of Alzheimer's disease. Later as the cranial kudzu intertwined and clogged her brain, there was no longer the irate taunt of "You think I have Alzheimer's!" As the disease took away her language skills and choked such verbiage as "Alzheimer's," her replacement words were revealing, devolving into "You think I'm demented" or crazy, or even psycho. I felt like a coward for not confronting the A word, Mother's very own scarlet letter, but I sincerely thought such frankness would only make things worse between us.

Mother spoke with vitriol of the incident with Judy. "She really hurt me. Judy made that doctor's appointment behind my back. Then when I wouldn't go to the doctor with her, she and Buddy went to my doctor without me." The corners of Mother's lips surely turned down. "So my doctor made me come in and get blood tests and that other doctor got the blood tests to see if I have Alzheimer's. But anyway."

Knowing that none of that had happened, I feigned shock. "Really?"

"Yes, and then the doctor sent me the bill for the blood tests. $300!" Thankfully Mother's delusions were fleeting, and when she returned to lucidity I could breathe easier and find comfort in my denial.

"You sound upset," I sympathized, using skills from a graduate school counseling class.

"I am so upset. And now I'm not sleeping because I've been under so much stress in the last few years with Howard dying and I've never gotten over it." She sighed. "But anyway." Even though our Dad had died over fifteen years ago, perhaps she never had regained happiness after she lost him. But that didn't explain the time disconnect.

Mostly my cowardice about confrontation paid off that day with Mother, when she confided in me and admitted that maybe something was wrong. Ever the nutritional optimist, I had given her some herbal supplements to support brain function. She said, "I've been taking those memory pills you gave me and I'm doing better."

"That's good."

"You know, you girls worry too much about me."

"Yes," I agreed. "We do worry about you."

Then she told me the secret that had been grape-vining through the family phone calls. We knew about it because Aunt Donna Lynn had told Judy, but with instructions not to say anything to Mother about it.

One afternoon a couple of months earlier, Mother called my aunt. "Do you know where Howard is? I can't find him anywhere. He should be home from work by now. Has Howard called you? I'm sick with worry. I don't know where to look for him."

My aunt calmed Mother, who had been napping and woke up disoriented. My aunt explained that Howard had died a long time ago. Sadly, this happened several more times.

I was very thankful that Mother told me about "looking for Howard." I said, "Oh, you must've been feeling really lonely."

"I will go to that doctor, but I don't need Judy to tell me what to do. And thank you for letting me talk about this. I don't have anybody to talk to. Nobody takes my side." I accepted her words as descriptions of feeling alone, not of actual events.

We were at an impasse. We couldn't make her. Even if we had physically carried her into a doctor's office or an assisted living facility, she had the legal right and willfulness to turn around and walk out.

Emails were flying that summer between Mother's chief "worrywarts." From Bev: *I think Judy told Mother the truth that she didn't want to hear. Mother wants to serve, not be waited on. She doesn't like anyone to tell her what to do about anything. God help me, but I may have inherited those stubborn genes.*

This email from me could be seen as capitulation or despair. *I do not say this as the bossy, know-it-all sister, but I say this with a slightly broken heart. Our only choice may be to do things HER way. Honestly, there is nothing new about that: we always lived by her rules. The thing we have to face is that we are losing our mother and we don't know what to do about it.*

From Bev: *Hey women close to my heart. I want to thank you, Judy, for braving the hysteria of Mother. I got an inkling of what you must have gone through today when I called and awoke her from a nap (no, she never takes naps.) She was totally confused, couldn't really figure out who I was or what I wanted. After a few minutes of my trying to get her to understand about the appointment to take care of her outpatient procedure, she asked me, "Could we start again? Who is this?" When I asked her again about the appointment, she started talking about the "confrontation" that you had, Judy. I was running an errand, picking up a cake at the grocery store for an 8th grade graduation, and I tried not to get into the whole thing. She is so paranoid that we (the girls) are talking, that you were trying to get proof that she was crazy, that she was being treated like an object, not a human being.*

I'm thinking that we're going to have to have an intervention soon. I'm fast feeling like assisted living in Memphis is better than having her live alone. I'm going to try to avoid the controversies while I'm in Memphis, but I doubt that it will be possible.

This was all happening rapidly. In April I was in Memphis and had an encouraging visit. In June Judy was there and the conflict ensued. Bev went to Memphis in July. Mother's ankle was badly bruised and swollen, and Mother conceded she had fallen. Bev massaged Mother's injury with arnica cream and it began to improve, though Mother's walking remained unsteady. Bev was amazing with Mother. All with no fights and a light touch. She took Mother for a minor outpatient surgery, back to the hearing aid office, fixed her disposal, icemaker, and garage door opener. Then Bev made a notebook with information about Mother's doctors and exchanged phone numbers with Mother's neighbors.

Bev told us all about her visit in an email. *My visit to Mother was the best I've had in a long time. I don't know who or what had changed, but I'm sure it helped that she had the outpatient procedure and had an excuse to allow me to help her. I do think that your incident, Judy, has made her reconsider her relationships with us. At the point that she called me fat and I bristled, she said, "I can't have another one." I said "another what," and she mentioned the day with you and Buddy.*

One day during her July visit Bev sat with Mother at the long maple table where so many meals had been shared, eating pork chops and stuffing that Bev cooked. In an effort to keep Mother nourished Bev had loaded Mother's freezer with single-serving dishes of twice-baked potatoes, enchiladas, and yams.

"I put some of this left-over stuffing in the freezer, too, " Bev explained to Mother. They were eating on the magnolia plates. "I heard you liked the food Marilyn left in your freezer."

"What?"

Bev upped her volume. "I heard you liked Marilyn's black bean soup."

"The black bean soup? Oh, right. I invited my neighbor Margaret over and we had it for lunch," Mother remembered. Mother's make-up was uneven and badly applied.

"I want you to like my food like that," Bev kidded. "I want to be able to wear the t-shirt that says 'I'm mother's favorite daughter.'" Actually, Bev was working for the Turk Award, the highest honor Mother bestowed. "Sit down," Mother would offer after one of us had worked especially hard on some project for her. "You've been workin' like a Turk." We knew right then that we had pleased her. What a badge of pride to get Mother's Turk Award, deserving of a gleeful cell phone call to a sister, "I got the Turk award!" Very different from what we considered the "Bad Daughter Award," where one of us became the anti-heroine of Mother's stories. Judy had usurped that dubious prize from me.

Again, Mother complained to Bev about Judy and Buddy. Shockingly, Mother talked with her mouth full of food, in what used to be a punishable manners misstep.

Bev cautiously responded. "Well, I wasn't there, but I'm sure Judy's intent was to help you."

"Why do you take her side?" Mother rearranged her breasts in her bra, beginning to lose her inhibitions as AD trekked through her frontal lobes.

"The neurologist was going to check on your problems with your legs and feet not going where you want." We didn't know that Alzheimer's was encroaching on Mother's parietals and causing these physical problems. "And Judy wrote you that sweet note, begging for forgiveness. Just think about all the times Judy's come to take you to appointments and how she came and got you so you could stay at her house and see your grandkids."

"You don't know how much Judy hurt me."

Bev tiptoed through the conversational minefields with Mother, restraining herself even if she disagreed. She tried to soothe Mother as the anger rose.

Mother sneered. "Don't treat me like a child."

Bev raised her hand with the helpless gesture of an open palm, and Mother batted it down. Our shadows had stepped into a harsh light, not in cahoots anymore.

Bev emailed more details of her visit. *I encouraged her to get her neighbor to drive her on errands, but I doubt that's going to happen. She said that when she quits driving, she will move into assisted living. She says it will be boring, but she's going to find an assisted living place in Memphis. I can't imagine it being more boring than her current life.*

Bev took Mother to see our aunts and uncles. The aunts said they thought Mother was better and that they checked on her almost every day. For that we were grateful. We hadn't gotten Mother to agree to hire outside help, but we had tightened the circle of communication and awareness between Team Lou and Lou's nervous daughters.

Chapter 7

Y'ALL, WE HAVE A PROBLEM

"I got off the phone feeling so helpless and sad. Mother said she had been sitting there all alone worrying about the kids. Y'all we have a problem."

An email from Judy

October 2008

The early afternoon shadows had begun to haunt Mother. Bev emailed about a phone call they had. Knowing their habits I could almost see them both, multi-tasking through the conversation.

"How are you doing?" Bev asked in her loud-just-for-Mother voice.

"It's getting cold. Nobody sits outside in the afternoons," Mother explained from her navy blue lounger, the footrest elevated, mail stacked on the end table beside her.

"That's too bad. You don't sound too good."

"I'm tired and stressed."

"Stressed? Is something wrong?" Bev, never one to sit still, like Mother used to be, was folding laundry, the portable phone cradled by her shoulder, again like mother used to do. Mother's phone obsession began long before cell or even portable phones, her kitchen multi-tasking aided by an extra long phone cord. Her yellow plastic kitchen telephone even had an attachment on the receiver to lessen the strain of holding the phone to her ear with her shoulder, freeing both of her hands for cooking.

Mother sighed. "Well, life is just hard."

"What do you mean?" Bev asked. In my imagination Bev walked down her hallway with folded laundry. She did that often during our sisterly phone visits.

"I'm not able to sleep at night. And you know I can't nap during the day."

Bev put the clean clothes on the bed. "You napped when I was there."

"I never nap. Why do you say that?"

"I'm sorry. Is there anything I can do for you? We still want you to come to the west coast for part of the winter. Spend Christmas here at my house. Judy wants you to visit her too."

"Not after what Judy and Buddy did to me. They told the doctor I'm demented." Mother hesitated for a moment, halted in one her brain's cul de sacs. "But anyway."

Bev interrupted before the conversation went terribly wrong, wondering again how it all got twisted in Mother's mind. "I don't think that's what they said."

"I'm just not going to talk to you about that. Let's change the subject. You girls won't have to mess with me too much longer. You'll be rid of me soon." Mother often threatened Bev with her impending death.

Bev's email ended: *Mother's saying new things about how well she's done in her life; that's why she had all those jobs and positions. That's why she is still able to take care of things. That dad needed pushing, that he wasn't aggressive enough without her. I started wondering if I missed her years as CEO or that time she was elected to public office.*

Judy continued the email discussion: *First yesterday morning Mom called and she said she could hear me talking but couldn't understand. She finally heard "Thanksgiving" and said she hadn't been invited anywhere. She had been and we already discussed it. I was so upset by the end of the conversation that she said, just write me a letter.*

Judy explained more in another email. Around 8:30 that same night Mother called Judy a second time with a different question. "Have your kids gotten home?" Mother was probably sitting in her favorite room stuffed with memories. The small room held the big clunker of a television set on which Daddy had watched the 10 o'clock news, a single bed for grandkids' visits, Mother's sewing machine, a pretty little antique desk with caches of note cards and stamps, framed photos of smiling family, a big round clock that had hung on the wall in all our dens for decades, and a full closet of more sewing accouterments though Mother had given up sewing years ago. This room had morphed into a museum honoring Mother's past rather than a source of entertainment.

Judy asked what Mother meant about the kids getting home.

Mother said, "Your kids. They were all here today but they left before I got to say goodbye." All the lamps in the room were surely turned on, as well as the overhead fixture, because Mother obsessed about light.

Judy reminded her, "My kids don't live with me anymore. All four of them are adults with their own places, and they haven't been to Memphis. They're all at their own homes in Knoxville and Maryland."

Then Mother repeated that they had been there with her.

As they continued to talk, Mother could actually hear Judy; Mother said she wanted to go to Chattanooga for Thanksgiving next week, and Judy told her she would drive over to get her. After they had talked another five minutes Mother again said that the kids had been there and she didn't get to see them before they left.

In light of all this, we planned Mother's holidays. It was a first, Mother letting us make these decisions. She would go to Judy's for Thanksgiving, then spend an extended holiday season on the West Coast visiting both Bev and me. It came after months of strategizing about how to handle Mother's "lonesome" winter and her disorientation. Mother would be spending the most time with me, and I would accompany her on the flights across the country.

Bev, recalling my tendency to meltdown, challenged me. "I think you're over-estimating yourself."

"She's our mother, she's failing, and she needs us. We'll make it work," I countered. Much patience would be required, but I was in it for the long haul.

Emails were flying between anxious sisters. A reminder of the "problem" flashed like a neon sign when Mother called Judy the very next night. "Don't try to use the Exxon credit card I gave you."

"I only use it when I drive to Memphis. I wouldn't need it right now. But why not? Did something happen?" Judy was having dinner in a Chattanooga restaurant with her husband, Buddy, and another couple. Judy later told me all this in a phone call.

"I had to cancel it." Mother was probably slumped in her lounger as dusk thickened like gravy in a cast iron skillet.

"Because?" The restaurant vibrated with cutlery and waiters.

"I lost my purse. About a week ago. I looked everywhere but couldn't find it."

"Where was the last place you remember having it," Judy asked, setting down her water glass and covering her left ear to shut out the noise.

"I don't remember. I looked everywhere. Uncle Bill even came over and helped me look. We still couldn't find it."

Judy became alarmed. "Was your checkbook in your purse?" We knew it was nothing for Mother to have over ten thousand dollars in her checking account.

"Yes."

"What about your social security card?" I could picture how Buddy might have stopped talking to their friends at the table and listened to Judy's end of the conversation.

"Yes."

"So, your checkbook, your identification and your credit cards were in your purse?" Judy looked around the table, grimacing to Buddy.

"But I cancelled my credit cards. That's why you can't use the Exxon card."

"A week ago?" Judy was thinking about identity theft, about the money Mother and Daddy had worked so hard to save for their retirement. "Did you tell Beverly or Marilyn?" Probably wondering why something hadn't already been done.

"No, I took care of the credit cards. I only told you because of the Exxon card."

"Did you close the checking account?" Judy shook her head to Buddy's questioning eyebrows.

"It's okay. I took care of everything. Don't fuss at me."

Judy jumped in the car the next morning and made a mad, six-hour dash across the state from Chattanooga to Memphis. She found the purse immediately under a sofa cushion where Mother had "hidden it from the robbers." Erasing the Bad Daughter title, Mother was extremely grateful to Judy for finding her purse, and thanked her copiously. Judy also found that Mother had started another skillet fire, this time burning herself, and getting a visit from the fire department. Mother explained that the fire department "broke down" her door after her skillet fire set off the fire alarm. She stayed furious at the fire department about that incident. How dare they force their way in when she didn't hear them at the door, did not hear what was obviously very loud banging on her back door, or her temporal lobes couldn't interpret the noise. Probably smoke filling up the kitchen. We never knew the real details about that particular kitchen fire, nor of the other ones either. More of Mother's secrets.

An email from Judy about her trip to Memphis: *Then I said I wanted to go look at assisted living places, and we went and visited her friend Lucy in an independent living facility. I found out that prospective residents need a form filled out by a doctor to determine if the senior is able to do independent living or needs assisted living. The receptionist gave me two names of doctors that specialize in senior care. I told Mom & she let me make an appointment with the one closest. I will take her to the appointment and then bring her home for Thanksgiving. I found her this morning at 5:45 rocking fretfully in her recliner and she said, "How did I end up with this doctor's appointment? What if he is a grouchy, mean old man?" I reminded her of my talking to the lady at the assisted living facility, and then she remembered and seemed okay. I plan to call tomorrow and tell them not to cancel the appointment unless I call personally.*

So we can take the doctor's appointment as a first step to preparing for the move. I told her I felt strongly that when she returns from the West Coast it would be time for her to move. Y'all can try to convince her to move out there, but in my opinion, it will be amazing if we can get her to move somewhere in Memphis without forcibly tying and carrying her.

Judy was a force for accomplishments in those few days in Memphis. She bought a safe where she stashed Mother's social security card and important papers, took Mother to the bank and moved some of the money out of her checking account, and even got a closed-caption phone, still convinced Mother's hearing was the deterrent in phone calls. When Judy returned to Memphis a week later to take Mother for Thanksgiving, the safe was empty and all of Mother's important papers, along with a box of unwritten checks, were nowhere to be found. Judy gave up looking and packed Mother into the car for Chattanooga. Later out in Mother's garage after her death, much to my surprise, I would find all those missing-in-action papers and other important documents in the bottom of the freezer, hidden under layers of frost-bitten meat, in a Tupperware container, wrapped inside several layers of plastic bags. Mother was right: "no robbers" could've ever found them there.

From Bev: *If we can get her to agree to move out of the condo, I think we should give it our best effort to get her near to one of us. She won't like any of it.*

With all of these coming changes, we'll just have to Face it, she's going to be depressed and angry, but it's for her own good. We'll try the tender, cajoling way, but I doubt that method will work. Get some tough skin, girls!

So in fact it happened: the doctor's appointment and then Mother spending two weeks around Thanksgiving in Chattanooga with Judy. The kindly Dr. Powers was an expert on treating the elderly. Mother talked to him with fearful honesty; he said emphatically that she needed to go into assisted living near one of her daughters. He wanted Mother back for tests and gave her some Aricept, an Alzheimer's drug to improve memory and mental function. Judy made the next appointment for late January after Mother's return from the West Coast.

I made the plane reservations. It cost me an extra $20 to talk to a real person; money well spent. "One flight from Seattle to Memphis. I need two seats together on the flight from Memphis to Seattle. No, just one person going on to California. No, Søren's ticket is separate. But he and I need the same flight to California."

My tickets were designed for the flexibility of my generation, not my Mother's. I printed out our itinerary: Marilyn--Seattle to Memphis round trip, Mother--Memphis to Seattle where I would put her on a twin-engine Alaska Airlines plane to visit Bev in northern California. I would stay in Seattle until Søren's arrival, Cincinnati to Seattle. After a few days in my stompin' grounds, he and I would both fly into Mt. Shasta's startling horizon. We would spend the holidays in California with Bev, her husband the fly-fishing aficionado Mitchell, Taylor their daughter who was home from her first semester at UC San Diego, and the guest of honor, our Mother, the matriarch. Who wouldn't be scratching their head about that jig-sawed travelogue? I envisioned myself maneuvering through bustling airports and narrow aisles of planes with my mother and her limitations, my trepidation a reality check.

Thus, I flew twice during that winter of the Great Recession, Seattle to Memphis and back, the landscape below a slick, white terrain. What the investment guru Warren Buffet called an "economic Pearl Harbor" staged a fitting backdrop for our turmoil with Mother. The over-amped financial bubbles had burst, fizzled out like my denial. The real estate market took the worst hit, and the safety of home collapsed under foreclosures. Loss and contractions were everywhere as if the physical world reflected my emotional apprehensions. Shelter was elusive. I hauled my carry-on with my tiny toiletries through snaking airport lines, crying babies, and incessantly ringing cell phones. Everyone toted heavy luggage to avoid the new charges to check bags. There didn't appear to be enough of anything to go around. Everyone seemed to be needy.

Yet, I blessed the miracle of Bev getting Mother to agree to this convoluted trip. Mother had not been to our West Coast homes in at least five years. She no longer wanted to travel. In our childhood vacations Mother had outfitted the family for leisurely trips in the station wagon, passing peeled and salted apple slices to the backseat to quell sisterly bickering. In spite of count-the-cows-and-horses games, singing church songs, and staying in motels as we motored across the states, our younger Mother longed to be back in her home. There it was more predictable. There she had control. Despite seeing the grandeur of the Washington Monument and the magic kingdom of Disneyland, Mother's worldview barely extended beyond the parameters of her southern world. She preferred known territory, having all the answers and her table set for supper.

Life moved more swiftly in the new millennium, and airplanes sped us to our desired destinations. With only a day's travel we would have Mother in our care. We acknowledged the downside: Mother might be more confused away from her own environment. Nevertheless, it was unmistakable, maybe even to Mother, that she couldn't spend the winter alone. Bev and I dreamed that we could keep her longer, even permanently with us. Mother's Memphis contingency, Team Lou, applauded this trip. Verbally tiptoeing so not to criticize her behavior, they seemed ready for Mother to be looked after by her daughters. Team Lou didn't say it directly, but perhaps the responsibility had become too much for them.

Meanwhile, I called Judy and asked her about Mother's stay during Thanksgiving. Though Judy said everything went well and that they had a good visit, Mother had introduced herself to Laura, Mother's twenty-something granddaughter, whom Mother saw regularly. How very gracious of Mother, getting up out of her chair, walking over to Laura and introducing herself so that Laura would feel welcomed. In Mother's defense Laura came into the house with a couple of her friends. We accepted Mother not recognizing Laura as expected disorientation while we had her uprooted. We weren't aware of her neurons being choked to death by brain kudzu.

Air travel in 2008 was no longer the luxury of my parents' vacation in 1946 with pandering stewardesses. Now cynical flight attendants served food for purchase only, which did not include a custard dessert. On one flight I sat literally on the very back row of the packed super jet, wedged in the middle seat. I jammed myself into the sardine-sized space after stuffing my backpack under the seat in front of me, thus eliminating room to stretch my short legs. By the window was parked a man tipping the national scale on the obesity meter. Not that I would be so politically incorrect as to malign someone with weight issues, especially since I am not skinny, but his poundage oozed over our shared armrest. I fidgeted, nervously adjusting to his overlap and my dwindling portion of comfort. He failed to see my squirming as an attempt to be considerate. He frowned and said harshly, "Stop it! Just relax. It's going to be a long flight." Then, and I swear this is true, the woman beside me in the aisle seat, spread her legs, and in a preamble to knitting swirled her yarn in an expanding infinity symbol, her figure 8 movements around her knees contracting my other side. I shrunk further into my central cavern, vowing never to fly again. The man on my left was correct, it was going to be a long flight. However, most travelers were cordial. I saw strangers helping each other, heard a lone trumpet blowing a Christmas melody over the blaring announcements of flight departures.

Memphis, December 2008

We took an elevator up to the lawyer's office and waited in the lobby, where the perfume of towering flower arrangements layered our nervousness. Sweet iced tea would have been bland compared to the receptionist. I dressed in a tailored jacket and mid-calf skirt for this appointment with Mother's lawyer. Lately Mother had grown more critical of my style, telling me that I looked like a field hand. She was no fan of overalls, even at home. Overalls were country clothes. She prided her city sensibilities.

Mother had an old will, and everything would be equally divided between the three daughters. This was stated very generally: all money, real estate proceeds, and furniture into thirds. More current decisions were not in it: medical power of attorney and executor had to be addressed. We also needed a Living Will, to include a DNR ("do not resuscitate" decisions) and to put into legalese her end-of-life wishes. Mother had decided that I would be power of attorney, medical power of attorney, and executor. Other families divided the responsibilities, each offspring given a legal duty. If my having all the legal powers upset my sisters, to their credit, they never complained to me. As daughters we did not question Mother's decision and breathed a collective sigh of relief that resonated through our diverse geographies that these essential issues would be addressed.

There was nothing for me to sign at the lawyer's office, but we sisters thought it prudent to have a daughter there. I was counting on the lawyer's objectivity. What might be emotionally fraught for us, to a lawyer exists as a straightforward legal question. Thus, out came the standard form for end-of-life decisions. The lawyer left Mother and me in the large conference room, sitting next to each other at the long, lacquered table, to fill in the blanks: DNR, antibiotics, food, and water, all the questions of how she wanted to be treated at the end. Mother did not want to be kept alive by machines, but was unwavering about receiving water; she had heard that not getting water was very painful. I sat beside her and talked her through each question, trying to explain what it meant, what the outcomes might be. We were both tearful.

Mother surrendered, her voice cracking under the heaviness of the decisions and the careful opulence of the lawyers' office. "Just be kind."

"I was there with you when Daddy died, and I'll be there for you again." I touched her hand, her fingers delicate, her nails carefully filed, her veins as blue as her beloved hosta leaves. "I'll be kind and take care of you. I'll do what you want."

It required several trips to the paneled, high-rise law offices to get Mother's will updated. There was legal language to be fixed, along with the duties assigned to me. On the way home after one visit Mother, sitting on the passenger side of her gray Buick, started screaming, not saying any words, just yelling syllables. No warning, merely loud monosyllables emitting from my usually proper Mother.

Though strange, I kept my hands on the steering wheel, continued driving and said, "Well, that's a good way to get rid of tension. Just let it all out." And she did.

On Mother's dining room table set a stack of newly printed copies of a tribute to Daddy, a tribute I wrote almost twenty years ago when he died. After Daddy's funeral Mother had requested that I write something about him to put in her thank you notes. (Thank you notes, a very fine southern tradition, an evanescent art form.) I channeled Mother when I wrote the tribute, wanting to please her with the description of their life together.

She fixated on that reminiscence about Daddy. With her long-term memory compromised, she forgot that she had already sent it when Daddy died. Thus, Mother insisted on paying Laura, her efficient, organized granddaughter, to redo the tribute, old-school style. Mother mailed the original copy of the tribute to Laura, who put in on her computer and printed copies on antique-beige paper that she mailed back to Mother. In the matching envelopes that Laura included Mother sent the tribute in lieu of Christmas cards. Though it seemed weird to most of the family, I considered it the lesser of Mother's growing obsessions. She missed Daddy and searched for him when dead-ended synapses left her lost in a bleak time warp; in the stark absence of his jovial essence Mother longed for him. In deference, I only commented about the tributes, "How sweet." Later I believed she was sending it as her own obit, preparing for her imminent death.

Mother had already started packing her suitcase before I arrived in Memphis. I casually asked her about packing her meds, about the Aricept Dr. Powers had given her. She had stopped taking the Aricept: no, the pills didn't bother her; yes, it might've helped; no she didn't need it, she wasn't demented. No, she wouldn't take it! What would her friends think if they knew! End of discussion. My mother was not alone in this behavior; I heard similar stories from friends whose elders refused their AD meds.

I had planned to have no conversations in Memphis that would cause conflict, since it was the early phase of a very long visitation. I let subjects drop at the hint of discord. Mother, however, demanded often, "Do you think I have Alzheimer's?"

"I'm not a doctor," I said, sticking to my nutritionist mantra.

Mother's money and her control of it became a contentious matter around this time. While I was in Memphis we found out one of her bigger annuities had matured and she had the entire amount in her checking account. The woman who had problems with losing things, including her purse and checkbook, had a large percentage of her savings in her checking account. Naturally, all three daughters freaked about that. I again broached the subject.

Mother screamed. "I do not need any help with my money! I don't want you to touch my accounts. I've taken care of my money all my life and don't you dare think you can take over. Stay out of my business. I'll tell the bank not to talk to you. They love me at the bank. They know how smart I am. I know what I'm doing."

That was the only time she blasted me, and I softly begged, standing there in the home she loved. "Please," I said. "Don't yell at me."

Mother thought she had only put a portion of the annuity in her checking account. She claimed the woman at the bank advised her to do that when Mother had an overdraft while at Judy's during Thanksgiving. Only Mother explained it as, "I over checked my account." Aphasia and difficulty with daily tasks can be found on any list of Alzheimer's symptoms, a result of deterioration in the frontal and temporal lobes.

During this diatribe she told me that she wasn't making any more investment decisions. Like doctors, she was finished with the whole kit'n'kaboodle. Bev and I promised to keep a close eye on her checkbook and purse while she was with us. Would we glide around the house, setting the table or wrapping Christmas presents, with Mother's purse dangling at our elbow?

As daughters we knew these were major red flags. We had talked to her, but the subject of money was a source of mistrust for her. Granted, we were still trying to reason with her unreasonable brain. Her paranoia about us wanting to take, as in steal, her money was extreme. Laws exist to keep offspring from taking over parental finances, unless the elder agrees or some diagnosis proves incompetency. We accepted stopgap measures, relieved to have her covered for most of the winter. Once again to state the obvious, and at the risk of sounding pedantic, these financial decisions have to be made <u>before</u> there's a problem, before, before, before. When things are mostly all right, and some sort of sanity prevails. Banks and lawyers are trained to facilitate those decisions.

I watched Mother repack her suitcase for our trip. She wore a faded sweater and old slacks while lovely clothes hung her closet. I breathed deeply to relax and allowed us to become two girlfriends getting ready: oh, take that sweater, you look good in it, that'll be nice and warm, do you have enough socks? I watched her take everything out and put it methodically back in the suitcase two or three times. The next morning when we were ready to walk out to Alex's car to leave for the airport, Mother opened her suitcase at 6 a.m. in the middle of the kitchen floor, took out all of her clothes, stacking them in piles beside her suitcase, then repacked everything again, like a stuck "repeat" button. This was not normal conduct for Mother. She used to get ready for a cross-country RV trip with Daddy with much less effort. She could install a month's worth of groceries in the motor home, put sheets on the beds, and situate the maps of the North American highways by her shotgun seat, without hesitation. She was more than a partner in crime. She readied the movable feast. Mother and Daddy on the road to Alaska. All easier than getting her out the back door that cold December morning. Alex patiently held Mother's heavy aqua coat for her as she put her long arms into the sleeves, and we were finally on the way.

As soon as Mother and I got settled in the plane on the first leg of our journey, there was some seat confusion. Who was supposed to be sitting where? A congenial man nearby exchanged seats so that Mother and I could stay where we were. It turned out he was a magician. A true working magician, rabbit out of the hat kind of guy, traveling to corporate holiday parties to perform. But I saw him as a reflection of the enchantment covering us on the trip, plunked down next to us by the prayers of family and conjuring of my women friends.

Mother was a real trooper about the long day of air travel. It was like sojourning with a child, only a child knows the parent is boss. Mother resented help. However, we have all gotten a good laugh out of Mother thinking the plane was a bus. Although what weary traveler could dispute the comparison. When I showed Mother the clouds out the plane window, she said, "We must be really high up in the mountains for all that snow." Airplane disassociation could be one way to overcome a fear of flying. It worked for Mother. Through two long plane rides and numerous conversations she never oriented to our sky ride. She thought we were on a bus from Memphis to Seattle. Faster than the speed of light, that bus. She probably had some uncorrupted bus synapses, though. When I was in high school she had ridden on a bus as a chaperone for rowdy, singing teen-agers, Memphis to Colorado. I was sixteen, flirting madly in the back of bus, trying to avoid my Mother's prying eyes.

Still unaware of some of her disabilities because she hid them so well, I offered her a large-print book to read on the plane, from a series she had liked. She tossed it aside with "It's boring. The same story as before." I prayed again for tolerance.

Thankfully, I was compassionate and did not take any of her rants personally. How mature of me. I plied both of us with ignatia, a homeopathic remedy to relieve stress. It seemed to calm Mother. Although at the end of the day when I handed her more ignatia, she said, "I need something stronger."

Mother was good in brief encounters with strangers: charming and even witty. Between flights cheerful wheelchair "drivers" propelled Mother to our next gate. To one wheelchair person, Mother joked, "Do you have your license?" It reminded me of the night Daddy was in the hospital just before he died, and I went with him for some final, ghastly test. He asked the person who was pushing his gurney the same jokey question, with one of the last sparkles in his eyes. "Do you have your driver's license?" It was a bittersweet recollection, in the southern tradition of politeness to strangers.

In one layover, I sat Mother down and stepped away for less than three minutes to call Bev. When I got back to Mother, she had lost her hearing aid. I had seen her take it off during the "final descend." Soon there were about half a dozen weary travelers on their hands and knees on the dirty airport floor, looking for the tiny hearing aid, lifting up bags and old newspapers, tossing aside jackets and coffee-darkened styrofoam cups while Mother and I went through every inch of her purse. We unloaded a bewildering array of contents. Eventually Mother realized she had the hearing aid in her ear the whole time. The kind search team hid giggles.

"Don't tell anyone," Mother asked of me.

The act of flying with Mother from Memphis to Seattle, then getting her on a short, direct flight to Bev's must have given me some major good karma points to compensate in a world of dubious choices. Or maybe it was just pay back for Mother birthing me. After all, she almost died when I was born. The whole "almost bleeding-to-death" thing. Transfusions, the true maternal sacrifice. What's a little plane ride in comparison?

The local news called it "the Deep Freeze" or "December storms." Mother and I landed in Seattle surrounded by snow. I got her on a short, direct flight to Bev's and went to rescue my car from a coat of ice and snow, me *sans* gloves or scraper. The northwest was snowed in, picturesque and dangerous. Tired, I carefully maneuvered the ice-polished streets, avoiding the bridges, finding main thoroughfares with steep inclines already closed. I drove white-knuckled that night, close to home but in a city with no true snow plans. As I proceeded nervously and slowly, Bev called my cell from California. Bev and her husband Mitchell had collected Mother before I could get to my house, which normally took twenty minutes.

Snow, a rare event around Puget Sound as well as the South, shimmered gossamer and surreal. It would cover the landscape almost symbolically during this expedition with my mother, requiring extra protection against the cold, and trapping us in its perilous, silent splendor.

Chapter 8

THE SCIENCE OF TROUBLE MAKERS IN THE BRAIN

"My own brain is to me the most unaccountable of machinery--always buzzing, humming, soaring, roaring, diving, and then buried in mud."

Virginia Woolf

ALZHEIMER'S VILLAINS

As Alzheimer's disease manifests in the brain, nerve fibers around the hippocampus fray and become snarled, short-circuiting information transmission. Pathways are stymied as synapses are blocked. Scientists continue to search for the activation of this brain deterioration, unsure of the causes. Presently it is even difficult to distinguish between the source and the symptom.

Sometimes a natural function of the brain becomes problematic. These brain villains were not necessarily born bad, but they grew more threatening as they accumulated. While the body can be amazingly resilient and protective against invaders, the ominous gathering of brain troublemakers may eventually outflank even the strongest brain.

TAU TANGLES

Tau (rhymes with wow) has a job inside the brain cell: the twisted strands of this protein form a microtubule for transporting nutrients and other necessary substances.[1] When these tau cells die and are not removed, their frayed ends form tangles in the interior of brain cells. With this loss of tau structure, the intrastate cellular highway collapses, and the brain trucking system for eliminating waste and delivering important goods cannot get through the tangles. These tau tangles interrupt the business of the neurons inside the cells.

BETA AMYLOID PLAQUES

Beta amyloid plaque can be found in the fatty membrane surrounding nerve cells in the bodies of both healthy and unhealthy people because of normal tissue degeneration or oxidative damage. Scientists mostly considered amyloids a kind of brain garbage, which some brains discard more easily than others.[2] These amyloids, normal brain proteins whose role remains a mystery, are not especially toxic; however, new research with animals is investigating the hypothesis that plaque is also formed in response to infections.[3] "The brain's defense system rushes in to stop the invader by making a sticky cage out of proteins, called beta amyloid. The microbe, like a fly in a spider web, becomes trapped in the cage and dies. What is left behind is the cage — a plaque that is the hallmark of Alzheimer's."[4]

Mass accumulations or the clumping together of these amyloids impede function between the cells[5,6], turning plaque into one of the brain robbers. Since plaque is also implicated in heart disease, associations have been made between heart disease and AD, which may indicate similarities in the prevention and treatment of both. As in heart deterioration, blood supply is decreased by these blockages of beta amyloids.

Thus, beta-amyloid plaques become blockages in the brain, getting in the way of synaptic communication. Increased plaque deposits attract inflammation. As plaque and tangles increase, brain cells die, and the brain shrinks. In this case, size does matter.

Here is a perplexing fact: Alzheimers disease doesn't affect everyone the same. People with this brain physiology may have no behavioral symptoms. A 2008 study from brain autopsies showed brains with "significant amyloid burden" but those very people having died with sharp minds and perfect memories.[7]

INFLAMMATION

According to the Linus Pauling Institute, "Acute inflammation is a normal process that protects and heals the body following physical injury or infection. However, if the agent causing the inflammation persists for a prolonged period of time, the inflammation becomes chronic."[8] We recognize our body's immune system fighting off the microbe, bacteria, injury, or other unknown toxins by the signs of inflammation: redness, pain, heat, or swelling. Inflammation, once a Good Guy fending off infection, turns into a culprit when it becomes chronic. At that point it is associated with everything from pain to cancer, from depression to heart disease, and in every "itis" in between, such as bronchitis and arthritis.

The immune response is a complex system with many players, having cool names like complement proteins, TNF (tumor necrosis factor), and Natural Killer Cells. These immune players rush in to protect against damage. However, they need to be turned off after their job is done because they can also function as pro-inflammatory messengers. In AD, inflammation gloms on to the amyloids and tangles. The cruel cycle continues: healthy cells are attacked, and cell degeneration leads to more amyloid. Repeat chorus, an unwelcome dirge.

"It does appear likely that the inflammatory pathways of the innate immune system could be potential treatment targets," said Robert Moir, assistant professor of Neurology at Harvard Medical School.[9] Currently diet and nutrition are being studied as an influence for turning down these inflammatory markers.

STRESS

Cortisol (the official name being hydrocortisone) is released by the adrenal glands and has the commendable job of helping our body respond to stress. However, no one doubts that stress can be cruel. Like standing in long airport queues dragging unwieldy luggage, stress is an unavoidable condition for many in modern society. But when stress invades life, it can compromise our health and well-being by increasing the cortisol levels in the body, pushing this good fellow cortisol into outlaw land. There stress thrives, willing and able to take a shotgun and damage many of our body's pathways and processes. Cortisol can weaken the immune system by blocking T-cells from doing their job, [10] can increase glucose production, and is a factor in contracting blood vessels and raising blood pressure.[11]

Cortisol is also utilized in creating memory, evolving from the caveman days of "fight or flight." For early humans to survive, their reptile brains needed to remember the threat in order to avoid it.

(The bigger the sensation or fear, the stronger the recollection.) Therefore, cortisol assists epinephrine in making and storing memories in the hippocampus.[12] Sadly, too much cortisol, rather than facilitating memory, decreases memory retrieval and damages the hippocampus, causing cell dysfunction and even cellular apoptosis (cell death) in the brain.[13] Therefore, stress is a factor in a shrinking hippocampus, which is an Alzheimer's marker and thought to be an influence in its onset.

Recent mouse studies have substantiated the role of stress in increasing hippocampus levels of beta amyloids and tau tangles. It took only seven days of injecting mice with a hormone similar to human stress hormones to raise the beta amyloids in the mice brains by 60%.[14] Other studies found much the same results: stress can produce tau tangles and beta-amyloids globs.[15] A long-term study of about 800 members of a religious order revealed that the people most prone to stress had twice the risk of Alzheimer's.[16] In contrast, The Religious Orders Study found that "conscientiousness, an individuals' tendency to control impulses and be goal-oriented" was robustly associated with reduced risk of AD, MCI, and also with slower cognitive decline.[17]

Several years before Mother's symptoms became evident, she experienced a very apprehensive period about some business property. It was unfortunate, seemed unrelenting at the time, and she would not let us, her daughters, have any input about the situation. At the time I said to Bev, "That will take two or three years off her life." Little did I realize the truth of that remark.

Needless to say, stress is unavoidable. It is possible, however, to alter our reaction to the body's mental and emotional alarms. Mother was a worrier her entire life. She had infinite crosses to bear and those kept her awake through endless sleepless nights.

Sleep deprivation is another vicious cycle: not enough sleep leads to anxiety, while increased cortisol may make for a wide-awake night. Studies are now charting the link between sleep deprivation and Alzheimer's. Changes in sleep may precede cognitive symptoms in AD patients, leading to a strong association between disrupted sleep and the development of the disease.[18] It has been discovered that during the day, the waking hours, the levels of beta-amyloids increase, and at night, during sleep, amyloid levels fall.[19] The conjecture follows that during sleep the excess amyloids are removed. Sleep deprivation, consequently, reduces the amyloids' elimination.[20]

DEPRESSION

Not surprising, stress can beget depression. Elders who suffer from depression have about twice the risk of developing AD; [21] but because of the complexity of this association, questions remain. Is depression a symptom of dementia or does early dementia cause depression? Other researchers are studying whether depression or stress causes dementia, and if depression reduces brain volume.[22]

ADVANCED GLYCATION END PRODUCTS AND HIGH BLOOD SUGAR

Advanced Glycation End Products (AGEs) are compounds formed within the body when proteins or fats combine with sugar, especially high blood sugar levels. Or as a 2006 study explained, "Advanced glycation end products are modifications of proteins or lipids that become non-enzymatically glycated and oxidized after contact with aldose sugars."[23] They mess with your cells, and not in a cute way, and can accumulate, becoming pro-oxidant and pro-inflammatory. To further identify AGEs as ruthless: smoking causes AGEs.

Inside the body this complex reaction creates toxic molecules that cause local and systemic inflammation, release cytokines, and can lead to stiffer cells and premature aging.[24] It's a nasty little pathway: AGE formation leads to eventual accumulation, increased inflammation, oxidative damages and stiffened blood vessel walls. Diabetics are particularly vulnerable to AGEs formation. These advanced glycation end products can accumulate in memory areas of the brain, harming blood vessels along the way. AGEs have been found to be an event in the early stages of AD. They can react with beta-amyloids and promote those accumulations; [25] because plaques and AGEs are "in cahoots, sweet pea, they're partners in crime."

In addition, AGEs can come from the food we eat. Meats, especially fried, are high in AGEs. Tufts University, a leader in nutritional research, explained that AGEs are made outside the body when sugars are combined with fats and proteins during high heat cooking.[26] Think browning meat. Think grilling. Although in the South "Died from too much barbeque" would be considered a fine obit, I'm going to continue with this finger pointing. Think high fructose corn syrup and colas. Studies have found that "diet, especially the modern Western diet, provided a relatively large portion of preformed AGEs."[27]

These AGE compounds, which are everywhere in the body, can be removed during sleep. However, this removal is an easier process for the body if it's not flooded with AGEs. Unfortunately, as we get older, our bodies are less able to get rid of AGEs.

DIABETES

Blood glucose levels affect the hippocampus where learning, recalling simple facts, and Alzheimer's start. A small study published in 2013 of 141 subjects without pre-diabetes or diabetes looked at high blood sugar levels. High (but not diabetic) blood sugar levels showed lower word recall, while participants with low blood sugar levels scored high on memory recall.[28] Those higher blood sugar levels impacted the structure and the volume of the hippocampus.[29] Consequently, pre-diabetes (a range of higher than normal blood sugar levels but not in the diabetic range) is also a risk factor for AD. A 2013 study on blood sugar levels with over 2,000 participants found that even two months of high blood sugar levels led to 10% increased dementia risk.[30] My mother loved anything sugary, especially white chocolate, milk chocolate and Dove Bars. The sweetness comforted her taste buds but perhaps corrupted her endangered brain.

Diabetes, a disease where the body fails to produce or properly use insulin, stands out as a perpetrator in many diseases and is considered a risk factor for Alzheimer's disease.[31] Patients with Type 2 Diabetes were twice as likely to develop dementia as those without Type 2 Diabetes.[32] Though no clear path has emerged to establish the reasons diabetes might cause AD, the web of complex factors continues to be studied.

Diabetes damages blood vessels. This damage takes place in the brain as well as in cardiovascular disease (CVD). With impaired blood flow to the brain, vascular dementia may follow.* Strokes may be another cause of vascular dementia, as patients with diabetes have a 1.5 times higher risk of strokes, according to the Diabetes Association.[33]

A study of human and mice brains suggested that one explanation might be that a reduction of blood flow deprives the brain

---

* The Alzheimers Association states, "Vascular dementia is a decline in thinking skills caused by conditions that block or reduce blood flow to the brain, depriving the brain cells of vital oxygen and nutrients."

of energy. This lack of fuel can set off a process that eventually produces the sticky clumps of protein, which hinder synapse actions. Without sufficient energy, a brain protein and enzyme are changed[34] into an ingredient in the recipe for making brain taffy. Studies have discussed other links between diabetes and AD: Insulin resistance can also be found in the brain.[35] Insulin resistance hinders insulin from doing its jobs, one of which may be activating cell survival programs. Insulin might also reduce the toxicity of amyloids.[36] According to a 2015 study, insulin acts as a growth factor in the brain and is neuroprotective, activating cell regeneration and proliferation.[37]

For those with mild cognitive impairment, that danger zone between normal aging and dementia, diabetes and pre-diabetes "substantially accelerate" MCI into dementia by more than three years.[38] Depression strikes again and is sometimes associated with both diabetes and AD. Depression plus diabetes equals increased dementia.[39]

FOOD CHOICES

As a nutritionist examining this composite of brain robbers, I cannot ignore life style choices. Lack of exercise, smoking and less social contact have all been investigated as factors. The role of food and diet seems undeniable to me. The connections and causes of AD are complex and slightly unfathomable; however, my "Wanted" posters would include mug shots of soda pop, processed food, too much red meat, too much added sugar, artificial sweeteners and variations on that theme. Even when I wrote this I could hear my mother saying, "I can do without all the talk about sugar."

Chapter 9

A WHITE CHRISTMAS IN THE NORTHWEST

"Inching into exile, her mind has lost its hold. One touch and the whole tree comes apart."

Shawn Fawson, poet

December 2008

Bev's "Lou Report" from Lake Shastina, California: *Mom's been here 2 days now. No big confrontations yet. We did talk about her going into assisted living and she said, "I'm going to stay in Memphis. That's my home." She says that we chose to leave her a long time ago, that she's not that close to us really. But I'm taking her to Meadowlark, the facility near my work, tomorrow. She agreed to look at it, but didn't expect to have her mind changed. It probably doesn't help that we have 4 inches of snow on the ground and it's 11 degrees outside.*

She's already ready to be home. Help me out here. I tried to get her to watch a PG video, but my TV doesn't go loud enough for her to hear.

She needs a new hobby. We're going to the library where they have big print books, but she can't seem to sustain her interest in anything for very long. She likes the cats, but has asked me at least

8 times about where they sleep. I got her to work on Christmas arrangements. Give her some greenery and flowers and her natural abilities come out. Maybe we could get her to volunteer at a florist.

I "forced" her to take a shower today because she hasn't had one in 3 or 4 days, and we're going out tomorrow. I tried to get her to let me do her hair, but she wasn't interested.

She's had some trouble for several days with diarrhea. She ate the applesauce and drank the ginger ale I gave her then went to bed tonight at 8:30. I'm not sure that she's feeling that great.

Just when I think I can approach her like a child, she's insightful about the "insult." I think if she wasn't my mother, I could handle her like I would any forgetful, repetitive, sensitive elder. She has always been thin skinned, hasn't she? She takes offense and I don't even know it. Her talking patterns are full of circuitous comments that are just fillers. Sometime she finishes talking and I'm not really sure what she was trying to say. And then, of course, the next minute she's clear as a bell.

Mitch's asleep on the sofa. Tay's downstairs in her room. I'll go check on Mom in a minute. I do often, turning off lights and removing magazines from her hand. She admitted that she left lights on at home because she lived alone and was afraid. She had her room here dark last night after leaving a lamp on Sunday night, so she must be feeling more secure.

Bev's email about Mother reads like a real-time concentrate of Alzheimer's symptoms: constantly repeating stories, personality changes, increased stubbornness, hygiene issues, loss of comprehension in reading or watching television, and bowel incontinence. At the time, though, we didn't see Mother's behavior as expressions of AD; we were, in Mother's vernacular, beating our brains out to figure out what to do next.

Mother and Bev talked over coffee, looking out at the family of deer camped under the trees in Bev's yard. With Bev taking vacation days to be with Mother, they talked nonstop, a pastime our chatterbox Mother loved. Bev would bring up new topics but Mother eventually got back to not wanting to change her living arrangement.

Mother told Bev, "Alex said I could live alone longer."

Bev, having given up on a conflict-free zone, retorted. "Well, he told us that he thought you should move near one of us. And that's what everyone says."

"Who?"

"The aunts and your neighbors."

"You're going behind my back?"

"They called us. Everyone is worried about your safety."

After Bev took Mother to visit Meadowlark, Mother said it was the nicest retirement home she had ever seen. Though over toast and scrambled eggs the next morning, Mother switched her opinion, "It was just a bunch of old people sitting around." Bev sighed and wondered how they would get through the day.

Then re-enforcements arrived for the Mom crusade. Bev collected Søren and me at the airport in Medford, Oregon. We drove into northern California over the Siskiyou Mountains toward Mt. Shasta, which John Muir said, "Was as lovely as God and white as a winter moon." Bev and her husband Mitchell, hosts extraordinaire, went over-the-festive-top, a house lit in beauty, with an abundance of color and presents. Mother ceremoniously put the first ornament on the Christmas tree, and we all clapped and cheered the joyous occasion. The tree was topped by the recession angel with the broken wing; she had no health insurance. Everyone but Mother wore Christmas headgear: elf or Santa hats, reindeer antlers, and Søren's head was graced by the fuzzy white angel halo. Angel Boy, I called him.

We ate with the enthralled abandon of a hound dog on a coon hunt. Even Mother was impressed there in carnivore heaven. The younger generation, Søren and my niece Taylor, won the nightly card games or Mexican Train dominoes. Mother truly seemed to enjoy herself when we were all together. It was practically a Norman Rockwell painting, and we were elated to get to share it with our Mother, all the Christmas rituals and holiday music in a glossy white Christmas setting.

Mother, Søren, and I waited for our departure back to Seattle in the small-town Medford airport; because of more bad weather Bev, Mitchell, and Taylor had kissed us good-bye and driven back to Lake Shastina over the snow-slippery mountain pass. It was noisy and over-heated within the concrete walls of the crowded airport. Grandmother and first grandchild Søren, now a grown young man working on his PhD, sat side by side in the busy airport. "So, what do you want to do when you graduate?" Mother asked with sincere curiosity. Søren answered her affectionately. I watched their conversation from behind my *New Yorker* magazine.

A few minutes passed: "So, what do you want to do when you graduate?" Mother asked again. Søren smiled and nimbly gave the exact same answer.

Another few minutes. "So, what do you want to do when you graduate?" He never lost patience. Same composed answer, exact same words. It happened again, same query, same kind response, and then, as people boarded their flights, we moved to sit in another part of the airport, closer to the gates.

"So, what do you want to do when you graduate?" Mother asked Søren earnestly as we resettled. Søren never flinched and repeated the same answer.

Mother got up to go to the restroom, and Søren sat down by me. I smiled at him and deadpanned, "So, what do you want to do when you graduate?" We both cracked up, acknowledging Mother's genuine interest in him and the impediment of her stuttering, stumbling brain.

In the Seattle airport, Mother and I kissed Søren good-bye as he boarded a flight to Cincinnati, then she and I took a cab to my little cottage in West Seattle. At my house I claimed success with Mother by adhering to the family tradition of, as Mitchell called it, coddling her. Like the inked route across the creased state maps, Mother's emotions were always our guide. On childhood family vacations she cried to go home. Despite what the other four of us in the car wanted, Daddy would wipe her tears, turn his hat around on his bald head, put pedal to the metal and drive across state line after state line, stopping only for bathroom breaks and gas. But considering all the work required of Mother on those road trips, the picnics supplied, the Pecan Sandy cookies passed to fractious kids in the back seat, the clothes to wash, no wonder Mother got homesick. Also, hysterical Southern women have historically ruled with their histrionics, a talent modeled for generations and often indistinguishable from Alzheimer's.

Bev emailed: *My blessings are with you, Marilyn. I hope that you can find ways to keep Mom entertained and comfortable while working, dealing with the employment issues, and taking care of all of her needs. I would have had trouble if I had been working and didn't have the help of Mitch and Tay. That seems like a huge amount of pressure on you. I made it clear to Mother that I think that she needs to move very soon. Judy told her she had to move in February. It upset her, but we can't pussyfoot around this issue anymore.*

Mother would be with me in Seattle for almost a month. Along the narrow lane where I lived, no streetlights interrupted the inky night. The green belt below my home echoed with fireworks, long after Mother and I were in bed. We had quietly welcomed in the New Year with some combination of me cooking foods Mother liked while she perused the pile of magazines my friends contributed for her stay. My sisters and I were glad to see Mother putting on a little weight; she seemed healthier than when we started our Winter Home Tours in November, not as thin. We had worked to fatten her up at our houses, to give her body nutritional support and resources. However, when Mother did return to Memphis she told everyone that we didn't feed her. "Look," she'd demonstrate, holding out the waist of her slacks. "I lost weight. They didn't feed me. I had to pull my belt tighter, because my waist is smaller." We all laughed about that, since seeing was disbelieving. In reality we catered to Mother's tastes when she sat down at our tables: waffles for breakfast, cornbread stuffing, canned tuna (sustainably caught, of course) with boiled eggs and sweet pickle relish, and steaks "like buttah."

"Do you think she remembers to eat when she's in Memphis?" was asked during a sisterly phone call. "I'm not really sure she can cook anymore."

"She says it's not fun to cook for just one person, too much trouble." We wondered if she could handle those familiar kitchen chores. Once her literal daily bread, her frontal lobes could no longer follow the sequencing required in cooking and found meal planning too complex.

"Well, Sandra leaves food on Mother's back gate several times a week." Sandra, Alex's wife was a sterling cook, making southern dishes Mother loved.

"And Mother takes that food to her neighbors!"

"Old habits die hard."

"You don't need to be a nutritionist to know that you've got to feed the body to nourish the brain. Some greens would be a good thing." Another nutritionist outburst. "I'm not lecturing BUT, Pringle's instead of lunch, not healthy for a long list of reasons; milk chocolate bars for dinner, where's the protein in that?" Preaching to the converted, once again. Thankfully the sister choir was tolerant and liked to sing along.

Every room in my small house wore pieces of Mother's history: Papa Vinson's desk in my office, the 1946 Philco radio in my living room. One day I found Mother sitting in Mama Mat's rocking chair, looking at my vanity with the tri-fold mirrors, motherly paraphernalia spread on the surfaces like dusting powder of old. Mother pointed to a silver, mirrored box. "I got the silver box for Mama Mat for Mother's Day. It had candy in it."

"Candy came in a fancy mirrored box? Not flimsy cardboard?" I sat on the end of the bed.

"It was expensive, maybe $5. I was working at our store. Thomas came in and I tried to get him to get one for his mother, but he wouldn't spend that much money. He said it cost too much." Thomas was Mother's high school boyfriend.

Did my mother with her slumping shoulders look into my vanity mirrors and see herself in a gray Northwest winter or as a teen-ager with her Mississippi sweetheart? I could picture Thomas, tall like Mother, stopping in the store to flirt with her, but also like everyone else, he would be buying the day's larder.

"Granny Susie gave me that red sewing box," Mother explained about the small faded box she saw on the dresser. "Granny was sick, just about to die and she was in bed when I got to go in see her. That's when Granny gave me her sewing box. I was Granny's favorite." Little Willie Lou, covered again with the sweet icing of affection. What a dear gift given to my mother by her grandmother, a sewing box, carried for years from room to room, wherever buttons or hems needed fixing, wherever she was living. Mother told me about Granny's hard life. Her husband died soon after the birth of my grandmother Mama Mat, leaving Granny with three little girls and no money, no food stamps, no outside employment. "I don't know how they made it," Mother pondered. "I think Granny had to hire the girls out to work in other people's fields." Such trials. Mama Mat was definitely of hardy stock and lived with hushed determination.

"That's sad," I said. "Both Papa Vinson and Mama Mat lost their fathers early in life." My daddy's presence was especially dear in that moment.

One day we shattered the pretense by visiting Kenney Retirement Community. The Kenney, only a couple of blocks from my house was, in my opinion, everything we would want in a retirement facility: large, bright, well-maintained with rose and vegetable gardens, a library, and complete services from independent living to acute care. They had activities, art shows, emergency care, and an available pretty one-bedroom with a balcony. "I could walk over and see you every day, if you wanted," I gushed to Mother. "Or not, if you needed a break from me." I pointed out all the stimulating factors, the travel exhibits of the residents, the puzzles and computers in the various lounge areas, and the kind staff.

Back at home everything went downhill. She sat in her favorite chair with the large red-leafed fabric, and I sat on the matching ottoman. I dove into the issues. She could be close and I could help take care of her, she needed to move, it was time. She was furious. She wasn't moving. She could still live alone, she didn't need anybody.

"But what happens when you do need someone?" I pursued.

"I have enough money to hire someone." She was deep in the cushions of the big red chair.

"You'd rather have a stranger take care of you than one of your daughters? We love you and want to be there for you." The fireplace was hot against my back as I carried on about loving her and taking care of her, hauling out all of our previous daughterly conclusions. The fight felt endless. I used my tranquil voice and expressed love, which in my mind no mother could renounce. "I love you," I said again.

Mother actually mocked me. With a distorted face, the voice of a fairy-tale witch, and flailing arms, she screeched, "I love you. I love you. I love you!" Like it was the worst thing on earth I could say.

I went into the kitchen and sobbed. Then I heard her groaning in the living room, her sounds guttural and eerie. I couldn't go to her. I didn't know what to do, and I couldn't stop crying. This vitriol from Mother had never been a part of our lives, it hadn't even been allowed, and now she was mocking me.

She eventually came into the kitchen where I was standing in a corner, leaning against the cabinet, weeping. She told me, "HUSH." Not the gentle "hush" of a mother soothing her young, but a command from across the tiny kitchen. We were both at a loss.

She said twice, "I'll just go home. I'll just go home tomorrow. I can be myself there!"

Not that I was without sin. I fumed, "Well, call the airlines and change your ticket," knowing full well she had no skills for such a task.

"You're hard," she condemned, rightly so, probably mentally erasing my Turk Award.

Mother and I stared across my miniature kitchen, regret suffocating us.

I offered. "People have fights. They learn to get through them."

"How?"

"We try," was all I knew to suggest, although I realized how paltry it sounded after the new threshold of malice crossed.

I was face-to-face with the bottom line. Mother was not leaving Memphis and she would pay a stranger to take care of her, rather than choosing her daughters. We daughters had played our best cards, but lost the bet, probably lost the game, too. I cried because of the mean things we said to each other, and because it was going to get uglier, getting her into assisted living. I thought about what my friends had done: one had told her Mother they were going to see a relative. Instead she had taken her mother, always a passive woman, to a nursing home. She left her Mother there, crying and begging. An upsetting scene that haunts her still.

I told Mother she was mean and didn't realize how the things she said hurt us, which made me the envy of my sisters. I was not proud of saying that, but Mother was not the only one at her wit's end.

The next day after our fight, Mother reverted to her native gentility, expressing appreciation and affection. Her softness was so endearing; the amicable face she showed to the massage therapist, or to anyone she'd never see again. At home there were daily diatribes. She would tell me I was ignorant. I let it go and waited for the return of her innate southern hospitality. Thankfully she maintained most social skills. Must be a southern woman's essence, like the damp air she breathed, the desserts she served with every meal, that charm she dispensed, the approval she desired. I envisioned that charm and her talent for praying aloud as the last of Mother's personality that would disappear into the avalanche of her disease.

I took Mother for a couple of massages to make her feel better. Therapeutic massages can allay symptoms of anxiety. She enjoyed the massages and sat down to write the massage therapist a thank you note. It took Mother several efforts to write what would previously have been a routine thank you sentiment; one of her original talents, putting words in letters, now evaded her. How upsetting to see the once prolific note-writer laboring tenaciously over a small thank you card, full of misspellings and scratched out phrases, the words lost in the amyloids. I was beginning to absorb the extent of her lost aptitudes: her cognitive reserves could no longer pull off the Big Cover-Up for the cells that were dead and gone. No wonder she kept saying how hard life was. Even the most routine habits necessitated much effort with little mental response.

I took Mother to the doctor because she needed her blood pressure medications and blood tests for her next visit in Memphis with Dr. Powers. We went to my friend from Bastyr University, Dr. Afia, a Naturopath and a cheerful, caring woman who spent way too much time with her patients to have a profitable practice. The three of us sat around a large desk, an artistic creation by Dr. Afia's husband. In true naturopathic fashion, Dr. Afia asked Mother about everything. When I disagreed with Mother's answers, Mother and I argued. Mother explained to Dr. Afia that she was stressed out because she had to sell the house all by herself. Yes, that house sale from almost ten years ago. Where was Mother's understanding of time? Her ability to articulate her thoughts?

On our next visit the blood tests showed that Mother had no thyroid activity, high blood sugar, high cholesterol, low B12, low vitamin D, and too much iron. Alarmingly, Mother's blood pressure was over 200. Dr. Afia wrote out prescriptions and talked to Mother compassionately. Looking back at the results of Mother's blood tests, I would take them all to correlate with AD. At that time I did not know that high glucose levels, high blood pressure, low B12, low vitamin D, and increased iron levels are all considered risk factors for AD. I did not understand those factors could decrease cognitive function and worsen symptoms.

Getting her prescriptions filled, Mother and I got into another silly fight. She had a new retort to our disagreements, a sarcastic "You win" before diving back into the argument. After several times of that, I finally said to her, "You win." That didn't go over well. At the pharmacy her credit card was declined. Concerned about how to pay for her meds, I never stopped to wonder why my mother, the most frugal woman I knew, had her credit card declined.

Later when she thanked me for spending my time to take her to the doctor (an all day affair) I said, "That's what daughters do."

She said, "No. It's not."

To cap off the day she said she wasn't going back to see Dr. Powers. I put that boiling pot on the back burner, knowing I'd have to deal with it in Memphis. However, Mother was right about Dr. Powers. His office called explaining that Mother's appointment was on Martin Luther King Day, the office would be closed, and the appointment needed rescheduling.

Meanwhile, Judy was making a master plan in Chattanooga. She created a spreadsheet with problems, options, roles, and solutions. I dreaded the clashes such necessities would bring, but Judy was thankfully persistent in wanting to stay ahead of the next, inevitable crisis. She divvied out goals and duties. I undoubtedly became the uncooperative sister at that point, but like Mother, I couldn't help my cantankerous self.

Chapter 10

THE SCIENCE OF REDUCING THE RISKS FOR ALZHEIMER'S DISEASE

"Eat food. Not too much. Mostly plants."

Michael Pollan

BRING ON THE POSSE!

The causes of Alzheimer's disease (AD) are currently unknown, without any reliable evidence that anything can prevent the disease or stop its progress. Still scientists search for ways to reduce the risks of AD and to slow the progress of the disease, especially during MCI and the early stages of AD. Thankfully, help awaits those who wish to slow brain decline and support cognitive function.

In Westerns, whether books or movies, the sheriff often deputized a posse and they quickly rode into action, horses galloping into the sun-bleached horizon, kicking up dust in search of outlaws. The brain needs deputies against its antagonists; it needs a posse as protection against the bandits stealing neural abilities. My crew will be rounded up from everyday sources, just like the deputies of the old West.

CONSIDER THE DIET AS A WHOLE

No surprise that my lead deputy would be food choices. No one claims a change in diet to be a panacea for preventing illnesses; however, nutrition is an important factor in wellness. A healthier diet has been associated in studies with slower cognitive decline and a lower risk of developing AD.[1,2] Looking at the diet as a whole gives a bigger picture of how the brain is nourished by food. An undernourished brain is a cranky brain that is prone to memory lapses. Food is fuel, and the brain is a greedy glutton. A small organ, about 2% of body weight, the brain consumes about 20% of daily energy intake. More specifically, the fuel required by the brain is glucose. Don't get me wrong here, not sodas or high fructose corn syrup, but glucose broken down from complex carbohydrates. Glucose supplied by fruits, vegetables, whole grains, legumes and nuts; not protein, not fats, but healthy carbohydrates.*

In a 2015 study Alzheimer's biomarkers (measures of the disease) were affected by diet: the markers moved toward a normal level in those who ate a healthy diet, while the biomarkers of those who ate an unhealthy diet moved in the direction seen in people with AD.[3] An international study with over 27,000 participants found that older people who ate a healthy diet (including more fruits and vegetables, nuts and fish) may be less likely to experience declines in thinking and memory over time.[4]

Another study found that "nutrition and dietary components and patterns have a plethora of anti- and pro-inflammatory effects that could be linked to cognitive function."[5] Healthy eating involves anti-inflammatory food choices, thus taking on the inflammation culprits. Broadly stated a healthful diet involves foods choices like

* While the brain has the ability through ketosis to obtain fuel from protein and fats, I prefer to leave that complicated discussion for others.

vegetables and fruits (can't say that enough), whole grains, nuts, legumes, healthy oils, fish, and only moderate consumption of lean meats and dairy. "What we eat should be whole, minimally processed, nutritious food – food that is in many cases as close to its natural form as possible," says Dariush Mazaffarian, dean of the Friedman School of Nutrition, Tufts University and adjunct associate professor of epidemiology.[6] However, if you are allergic to or intolerant of certain foods, eating those may cause inflammation. Choosing an anti-inflammatory diet eliminates food felons, such as too much sugar and processed foods that can raid the brain.

A twelve-year study from Harvard published in 2013 compared diets high in inflammatory foods -- sugar, too much red meat, and refined grains -- with an anti-inflammatory diet, similar to a Mediterranean diet. Those choosing more inflammatory foods had a 41 percent greater risk of depression,[7] the inflammatory marker measured in the study. Many diets come back to the same suggestions: salads, berries, nuts, less red meat, more fish, less from the center of the grocery store and more from the produce section. The point is to eat more from the healthy groups, and less from the unhealthy groups — with stricter adherence to this rule leading to greater advantage. The unhealthy groups include red meats, margarine, pastries, sweets, and fast food or fried food. When it comes to healthy food choices, it's best to outnumber the marauding, inflammatory food groups with a larger posse of anti-inflammatory foods. However, an anti-inflammatory diet approach appears to reap brain benefits even when adopted later in life—sometimes aiding cognition in as little as two years.[8]

Acronyms proliferate when it comes to diet suggestions, sometimes adding to the confusion. Is the MIND diet better than the DASH diet? While many people feel more secure with daily food inventories, calorie counting or other paint-by-numbers diets, I prefer the freedom of personal choice within nutritionally-rich boundaries.

ADVANCED GLYCATION END PRODUCTS

Consider advanced glycations end products (AGEs), which may accelerate cognitive decline and AD symptoms. First, lower your intake of added sugars to reduce AGE formation within the body. The USDA Dietary Guidelines advised that added sugar be no more than 10% of caloric intake or about 50 grams daily. The American Heart Association and the World Health Organization recommended 5% or approximately 25 grams of added sugar daily.[9] These suggestions do not include sugar inherently found in the fruits, vegetables (yes, even beets and carrots contain sugar) or dairy. And from my "natural" perspective, the studies I've read do not support switching to artificial sweeteners as a way to decrease sugar consumption. Animal studies have found that the artificially-sweetened diet can stimulate appetite and promote hyperactivity and insomnia.[9] Population studies have shown that people who regularly drink diet soda are more likely to suffer strokes and heart attacks.[10] Besides boosting insulin and reducing glucose tolerance, artificial sweeteners can alter the good bacteria residing in the G.I tract.[11]

By cutting down on added sugar, foods that contain AGEs will be reduced: ice cream, cookies, cakes and processed foods. Also high in AGEs: bacon, red meat, hard cheeses and high fat foods like butter or mayonnaise. Lowering dietary ingestion of AGEs equates to less AGEs in the body. All is not bad news. Only 10%-30% of AGEs from food are absorbed into the body, [9] allowing room for some guilty pleasures.

Cooking methods greatly increase AGEs in food, especially high heat cooking, frying, grilling, roasting and broiling.[10] There are simple fixes: shorter cooking times, low heat, added liquid or steaming. An acidic marinate, like vinegar or citrus, acts to diminish the AGEs created in cooking meats, where sugar would greatly increase them.[11]

Though more studies are needed to verify this fact, antioxidants, especially vitamin C, may help to remove AGEs from the body.[12] Proudly wearing the badge in the vitamin C posse would be bell peppers, papaya, broccoli, and your favorite citrus fruits. B6 has been shown to combat AGEs in the body, inhibiting AGEs at three different levels of formation.[13] Since some of the best sources of B6 are meat and fish, as a vegetarian (who eats sustainable salmon), I choose to supplement with B6 in order to have a strong enough B6 posse to carry out all of their responsibilities.

EAT BREAKFAST!

As a practical suggestion, eating a good breakfast is important in my version of a whole foods diet. Breakfast has been touted to improve mood, memory and calmness. A protein-rich breakfast may increase dopamine, a neurotransmitter believed to support mental acuity.[14]

Green tea in a morning routine can add more antioxidants than some individual servings of fruits or vegetables. Green tea (*Camellia sinensis*) contains polyphenols, especially the catchin EGCG (epigallocatechin), which is the most active ingredient in green tea. While green tea has been studied for conditions as diverse as weight loss and cancer, newer studies have found EGCG to be the most potent for neuroprotection.[15] In fact in 2005, higher consumption of green tea was associated with a lower prevalence of cognitive impairment in humans.[16] The polyphenols work in several brain functions: fMRIs (functional magnetic resonance imaging) showed that EGCG increases brain connectivity between the parietals and frontal lobes to improve working memory and performance in healthy subjects. The other good news is that EGCG participates in the creation of new neurons, or brain plasticity.[17] EGCG phenols are particularly useful against beta-amyloid plaques by interfering with the assembly of the plaques, inhibiting amyloid formation, and changing amyloid shape to prevent binding.[18]

The amount of polyphenols in green tea varies. Loose leaf green tea, compared to a tea bag of green tea, has the most EGCG.[19] The fresher the leaf, the more nutrients will be present in the leaf, and loose leaf tea is generally fresher. The leaves used in most tea bags are actually the "dust and fannings" from broken tea leaves. Though the convenience factor encourages the use of tea bags in daily rituals, those processed tea leaves have lost most of their essential oils. I'm not dissing tea bags, but again suggesting you know the source. Where was your green tea grown? Were the tea bags treated with chemicals? Hotter water and longer steeping increase the release of polyphenols when using tea bags.

While some studies used a green tea drink, most utilized standardized extracts. Each menstrum releases individual properties: consequently, green tea may be extracted with water, alcohol, glycerin, CO2, or some combination of these methods. Personally, I avoid extracts made with hexane or other chemicals. If you want a bigger bang for your EGCG buck, you may decide to supplement with green tea liquid extracts or pills, devoted deputies in the pursuit of amyloid plaques. Green tea may be the most potent source of

EGCG, but dark chocolate, the skin and seeds of fruits like blackberries, apples, cherries, pears, and wine also contain this flavonoid.

SPECIFIC NUTRIENTS MATTER

B Vitamins

When on an anti-inflammatory diet, include specific nutrients and foods to boost your cognitive strength. B vitamins have a busy role in the body. They break down proteins, release energy from carbohydrates for the brain and nervous system, and are needed for normal brain function and the conduction of nerve signals. The duties of B vitamins anchor the needs of the brain's functionality.

B vitamins can be found in leafy greens, whole grains and nuts. B vitamins have a team mentality and, if choosing to supplement with individual B vitamins, they will be better absorbed in the company of other B vitamins. After all, they are often found together in whole foods. Not only do B vitamins work better together, but a study of 250 MCI patients found that B vitamins needed higher levels of omega 3s to be effective against cognitive decline.[20]

Folate is crucial in the nervous system at all ages, but in the elderly folate deficiency contributes to aging brain processes and increases the risk of Alzheimer's disease and vascular dementia.[21] Add folate to your diet with legumes, broccoli, and papaya. Due to processing, canned beans provide much lower amounts of folate than a serving cooked from dried beans.[22]

According to physician and author Dr. Andrew Weil, "Vitamin B6 helps in the production of neurotransmitters, the chemicals that allow brain and nerve cells to communicate with one another, ensuring that metabolic processes such as fat and protein metabolism run smoothly."[23] Consequently, a deficiency of B6 may cause confusion, depression or irritability. Avocado, banana, beans, nuts and whole grains reign as vegetarian B6 stars.

Choline is a precursor to acetylcholine, the most prevalent neurotransmitter in the body, important for learning, sleep and motor function. Lower acetylcholine has been linked to Alzheimer's and depression.[24] A diet high in monounsaturated fats (like olive oil, avocadoes and nuts) can also lead to an increase of acetylcholine.[25]

One of the most basic cellular survival processes, methylation, require choline. Many of the signaling processes in the human body involve passing a methyl group (one carbon and three hydrogen atoms) to another molecule. Building DNA, exchanging signals in the brain, and detoxification in the liver depend on methylation. Deficits in this function have been linked to memory loss and cardiovascular disease.

Choline acts as a key partner in this process, along with folate and vitamins B6 and B12. If those B vitamin partners are not available in sufficient amounts to assure adequate methylation, choline can provide assistance and help assure that methylation continues.[26] Although not officially classified as a B vitamin, choline appears to share their team mentality. Look to eggs with the yolk, turkey, salmon, shrimp, lean meat, tofu, mushrooms, whey and cocoa as good sources of choline.

Vitamin D

Vitamin D regulates neurotransmitters, helps maintain cognitive functioning and may lessen depression. Vitamin D plays a role in many functions of the body. Vitamin D receptors live on cells throughout the body, waiting for vitamin D to attach to receptor sites and initiate the activities of the cell. These receptors are found in organs and tissues such as the brain, heart, muscles and immune system.

Studies with mice found vitamin D may reduce the plaques associated with Alzheimer's disease.[27] A severe deficiency in D was associated with a 125 percent increased risk of dementia and 122 percent increased risk of AD, surprising even the researchers. This study followed over 1600 people aged 65 and older for six years.[28]

Selenium

Selenium is known to protect fatty acids in cell membranes from oxidation. Studies have found that a deficiency in selenium is linked to anxiety, irritability, depression and decreased cognition.[29] Although selenium's function in the brain is unclear, when the body is deficient in selenium, the brain is the last place where selenium levels drop.[30] It seems the brain holds on to selenium because it needs it. Sources of selenium are nuts, especially Brazil nuts, as well as pork, cod, tuna, mushrooms and whole grains.

ESSENTIAL FATTY ACIDS (EFAS)

While a comparatively small body organ, the brain is the fattest. The brain is composed of about 60% fat, making fats an integral part of brain structure and functioning. Therefore, the brain needs fats and works better with good fats rather than saturated fats.

If we are what we eat, then we can be potato chip brain or omega-3 brain. Omega-3s are long chained, essential fatty acids (EFAs) that the body cannot create; thus, they must be gotten through diet or supplements. DHA (docosahexaenoic acid) is the 22-carbon chain omega-3 making up about 20 to 30 percent of the brain. DHA is one of the building structures of the membrane phospholipids of the brain and necessary for continuity of neuronal functions.[31] It's critical for neuronal signaling and cell messaging. The 20-carbon chain omega-3 EPA (eicosapentaenoic acid) supports the anti-inflammatory pathways in the body, buttressing protection against chronic inflammatory conditions. Salmon and other fatty fish provide fully formed DHA and EPA. ALA (alpha-linolenic acid), an 18-carbon chain omega-3s from plant sources, can be converted to DHA and EPA by a healthy body with the aid of vitamins, minerals and enzymes. The rate of conversion, however, is low, and the percentage contested by experts. Vegetable oils, nuts, especially walnuts, flax seeds, hemp seeds and leafy vegetables offer ALAs. You need to eat a lot of them!

FOOD FOR THE BRAIN

Recall that new neurons are created in the hippocampus. We need those new neurons for a healthy brain and to protect against memory loss and other AD damage. Studies promote the role of nutrition in hippocampal strength. One study concluded that "modulating adult hippocampal neurogenesis by diet could emerge as a possible mechanism by which nutrition impacts mental health."[32]

All omega-3 fatty acids are concentrated in the brain, but DHA especially has been confirmed to promote neuronal growth.[33] A review study in the Journal of Nutrition stated, "DHA appears to slow pathogenesis of AD, acting at multiple steps to reduce the production of beta-amyloid peptide, and may help suppress neuroinflammation."[34] DHA also increases BDNF, the fertilizer of the hippocampus.[35] Higher levels of omega-3s in the blood stream were linked to 2.7 percent larger volume of the hippocampus.[36] A bigger hippocampus is linked to less neuron loss.

Flavonoids give color to food and are celebrated for their antioxidant, anti-inflammatory and cell communication properties. George Mateljan, founder of the non-profit World's Healthiest Foods, wrote: "Flavonoids are one of the largest nutrient families known to scientists, and include over 6,000 already-identified family members."[37] Specific flavonoids arise from particular plant colorings, and like any color wheel, hundreds of flavonoids (or color shades) exist in a single food item. Flavonoids in plants combat environmental stress and attract pollinators with their color; these survival skills of plants are passed on to the human body where they modulate signaling pathways.[38] Those polyphenols in green tea? Flavonoids!

According to my thesis, blueberries can be seen as a microcosm for examining flavonoids and whole foods diets.[39] Flavonoids in blueberries and other purple or blue foods, anthocyanins being the most significant, protect the hippocampus and stimulate new cell creation. These anthocyanins — also in cranberries, black beans, grapes and foods in the blue color spectrum— pass through the blood-brain barrier to optimize brain function.[40] Studies have shown that blueberries could improve short-term memory in all demographics.[41] Those studies were done with participants eating at least a cup of blueberries five times a week. Most benefits require therapeutic doses of these healthy foods. If you balk at blueberries everyday, include another anthocyanin-rich food in your diet, something tinged with purple like blackberries, figs, red onion, black rice or purple carrots.

Blueberries put me in my happy place. Big fat, sweet, azure orbs. Can't you feel those anthocyanins knock-knock-knocking on your hippocampus door? I love stirring them into soft goat cheese (local goats do it better). I add basil or spearmint from the garden and after a Zen moment of chop-chop, drizzle with a taste of raw honey. (Local bees also do it better.). Why on earth would Eve give it away for an apple? Surely there were juicy blueberries waiting for her in Eden. It was paradise, after all.

Excessive intake of bad fats and added sugar may negatively impact the hippocampus. Rats fed junk food had weakened hippocampal function, while antioxidants lowered oxidative stress in the brain.[42] Reducing calories also increased the hippocampal health of mice. One study claims that reducing calories may be as effective as exercise for hippocampal strength.[43] My conclusion? Choose whole, nutrient-dense foods rather than calorie-dense, processed foods.

THE GUT-BRAIN AXIS

The body is populated with bacteria, presently estimated at ten times the cells in the body, and 100 times the cells in the gastrointestinal (GI) tract. Gut flora are beneficial to the host organism, better known as the human body. In stores these "good" bacteria are sold as probiotics.

The GI tract has been called the body's second brain. The gut has its own independent nervous system and is the location of hundreds of neurochemicals the brain needs to regulate mental processes such as learning and mood. This gives new meaning to "I had a gut feeling." More than just mental tasks, these neurotransmitters — with such names as GABA, serotonin and norepinephrine — carry messages that affect everything that goes on in the body, linking the brain and spinal cord with muscles, organs and glands.

Microbiome research is in the early stages and includes MRIs to link microflora with brain activity and behavior changes. "I do believe that our gut microbes affect what goes on in our brains," said Dr. Emeran Mayer, co-founder of the UCLA Collaborative Centers for Integrative Medicine.[44] Now scientists see the interaction between the GI tract and the brain as a two-way highway, where bacteria may be directing the brain, via the Vagus Nerve.

Researchers believe that gut flora use neurotransmitters, such as serotonin, to send messages to the brain. Dr. Mark Lyte at Texas Tech University Health Sciences Center saw neurochemicals not described before being produced by certain bacteria. He said, "Bacteria in effect are mind-altering microorganisms."[45] Those good bacteria get tiny, tiny little deputy badges for their work in the hippocampus.

Adding probiotics to the diet can be as easy as eating yogurt, kefir, sauerkraut, kimchi or other fermented foods. Many flavors of kombucha drinks are available. Besides increasing probiotics in our diets, recognize what decreases the colony of good bacteria: antibiotics, stress, illness, GI tract inflammation and too much alcohol. Be kind to those supportive allies in the gut. Feed them the fiber they need, from fruits, vegetables and especially the fiber inulin found in such foods as sunchokes (aka Jerusalem artichokes), bananas, onions and garlic.

THE IMPORTANCE OF SLEEP

"Sleep is such a mercy," writes Marilynne Robbins in Lila.[46] During sleep the body actively rounds up the brain robbers in nightly raids and removes them from the scene of the crime. Sleep allows the body to heal; amyloid plaques and AGEs can be removed. But sleep can be elusive, whether because of AD damage, a stressful job or staying too late on the computer.

Serotonin has been researched for the regulation of sleep and was found to "modulate circadian rhythms, sleep and waking."[47] While a variety of neurotransmitters are produced in the gut, a whopping 95 percent of serotonin, the feel-good neurotransmitter, resides the gut.[48]

Tryptophan is an amino acid that converts into 5-HTP, which becomes serotonin. Contrary to popular belief, tryptophan is the least abundant amino acid in food. (No, it's not true that turkey induces sleep with a load of tryptophan.) To turn tryptophan into serotonin requires B6 (a busy, busy B) and niacin working with complex carbohydrates, other amino acids and enzymes. Vitamin C and D play a role, too. Again, nutrients work best in combination as supplied by a diet of foods as close to nature as possible. This pathway can also be enhanced by experiencing early morning light outside. Some building blocks for serotonin include bananas, beets, brown rice, fennel, fish, milk and legumes. 5-HTP, the intermediary step between tryptophan and serotonin, is available as a supplement and sometimes is taken to aid sleeping.

Natural sleep remedies abound. Here's another shout-out for vitamin D. One study found that for the elderly, higher D levels were linked to more hours of sleep per night.[49] Some people find that melatonin assists with sleep. The catch about melatonin: it can help you fall asleep, but it doesn't help you stay asleep. Herbal botanicals may offer assistance with sleep. Valerian is an herbal muscle relaxer, while skullcap, holy basil, kava and passionflower have been used to combat a restless mind.

With most problems, solutions don't exist in a quick-fix pill. Solutions require lifestyle changes, a commitment to wholesome eating, time and forgiveness. Rather than dwelling on the no-no list when improving your diet, emphasize the positive additions. (Ah, channeling my daddy again.) More kale can crowd out fries, quinoa can fill in for red meat. Gradually the food on your plate can shape shift, even if only once a day. Habits evolve as your life transforms, and perhaps your brain clears out some kudzu along the way.

Chapter 11

MEMPHIS MELTDOWN

"The river is brown and glossy, shining like the brown-glass of old bottles. Here at Memphis it is almost a mile wide; you can barely see across it. The Hernando de Soto Bridge arches into Arkansas, into oblivion, carrying lines of brightly colored cars like so many little beetles. Light glints off them like thousands of tiny arrows."

The Last Girls *by Lee Smith*

Memphis, January 2009

Mother and I returned to Memphis in late January, and she couldn't get her luggage fast enough. I couldn't help but tease her. "That's all you could talk about, getting home. I thought you might kiss the ground when we got here."

"I might," she agreed as we stood side-by-side, survivors watching the baggage carousel make another empty circle.

Because Mother couldn't wait to get back from her West Coast visits, I assumed the South would be her balm. However, her inabilities to handle normal activities crushed her, and she reacted like the control group of caged mice in those studies I continually quoted.

Mother greeted me with dysphasia on Friday morning, the day after we flew back into Memphis, a day of bickering and car trouble. "My conscience told me the car wouldn't start." I reached into her cabinets for the essentials to brew green tea. It was my fault that Mother couldn't handle the daily realities of her life. Or so Mother perceived, blaming whichever daughter was in her space at the moment. According to Mother, "Y'all just take over and I've always taken care of myself!" Though that hardly seemed the case, the contents of her billfold flung across the cabinet top, while her '93 Buick sat comatose in the garage.

After several disagreements between Mother and me, I got AAA out to her crowded garage to start her car. The nice young man patiently explained the problem. Mother fretted and called her neighbor. When the neighbor recommended a particular mechanic, Mother disregarded the advice of the AAA guy whom I preferred. Clearly, the neighbor was a man and I only a female. When the recommended mechanic didn't "roll out the red carpet" for her, Mother railed her disappointment as I drove us home in the aging LaSabre. That mechanic cost $30 more than the AAA price. The heat in the car blasted, as we drove past a fountain frozen solid in icy incongruity.

I took a short walk to regroup, but I shivered against the winter chill. Unlike Seattle, busy street corners did not proffer the coziness of coffee havens.

Mother called my cell several times. "Where are you? I woke up and you were gone. I thought everybody had left me." She sounded distraught.

Judy called me before I got back to Mother's. She had talked to Dr. Powers and he was 99% sure Mother had Alzheimer's. Her symptoms fit all the descriptions. I stood outside in the freezing weather beneath the bare limbs of an old oak talking to Judy, trying to disseminate all the bad news. Once again my hands were without gloves, as I tucked one at a time into my coat pocket.

The next day, basically against her will, I took Mother to get a new television. She protested. "But I have two TV sets!" Her mouth tight and fierce.

"Old as the hills and almost as big," I thought, but only tendered, "But neither of them work."

My sisters and I imagined the constant hum of television might console Mother, since that sound had been Mother's companion for most of her life as she sewed or did her chores. Much like the dream of the hearing aid solving her communication problems, we sisters looked to yet another appliance for relief. The familiar sound of television would surely quell the fears shouting in her head. I clutched the big steering wheel of her ole gray mare of a Buick, slowly taking the curves of the wide Memphis avenues.

Mother challenged, "Do you think I'm off my beam?"

"Do you really want to talk about this now? I think you have some memory issues," I allowed, as always avoiding the suggestion of Alzheimer's disease. "Let's not talk about that now. Are you sure we're going the right way?"

"You undersell me!!" she yelled.

I took a deep breath and summoned my last bit of endurance, like licking my finger to collect the final crumbs of corn bread. I navigated my hometown streets, which I had left forty years before. I had no idea where we were.

"Why did you say I had mental problems?"

"I didn't say that. I said you have memory issues."

"Why did you say that?" she demanded shrilly.

"Because you asked me. I said I didn't want to talk about it, but you kept asking."

Mother sneered, "And you were such a model child."

We survived the catastrophes of the day. After driving her to get the car fixed and doing other needed errands, she thanked me profusely.

"No problem, daughters are happy to help take care of our mothers," I reassured her.

"No, not daughters." She stared out the front windshield at her neighborhood stop sign. "I should've had sons. Or I should've remarried after Howard died."

I clinched my teeth and kept my eyes straight ahead.

It was most heart wrenching when Mother and I were caught off guard by her confusion. Sitting in her living room together, I explained again that we got her prescriptions filled in Seattle because she was out of them. She spoke hesitantly, "I didn't know I was going to Seattle."

Every night in Memphis she would appear at my bedroom door, her shoulders hunched over in her new Christmas pajamas, her white hair flat on her head, blurry in her sleepiness. "Can I get you anything?" was more of a request from her, a mantra of motherhood. For a moment there was nothing threatening between us, just mother and daughter, wishing the other a good night's sleep. The kindest that life had to offer. Then she'd ask, "Are you warm enough?" the heat up to 80 degrees, me on top of the covers.

Obama was inaugurated while I was in Memphis. Millions of people were in D.C., joyous, excited, and hopeful. As the Obama family rode the train to D.C., crowds gathered all along the way, waving and cheering. One reporter, when queried about the unprecedented outpouring, replied, "It shows the depth of their despair." I could understand that; I felt mighty desperate, too. We all needed hope. If waving to our first African-American president along a railroad-less-traveled could have altered our family's course, I would have been there, waving brightly, praying loudly.

I treasured Mother's rarified prayers over every meal, the language of religion floating above the thickness of brain damage. Back in Memphis, she never finished the small amount of food she put on her plate. Instead I found a trail, unbecoming my fastidious mother, of milk chocolate candy bar wrappers throughout her home, tossed beside her bed. To my relief we didn't fight all the time, and she even complimented my hair, often a point of contention. On my last night in Memphis she asked me if I couldn't stay another day or two. Quickly, she took it back because she wasn't going to tell us she was lonesome or stressed, since we reminded her of such words to reinforce our campaigns.

Mother got mad at me when I called the phone company to fix her overdue bill and stop the collection company from badgering her. She pounded the counter top. I was startled by the ferocity. In the glory of hindsight I can see how that terrified her, that I completed the menial tasks she couldn't even start.

"I will NOT have you taking over my life!" she screamed, sitting beside me, envelopes and old bills scattered on the cabinet top. Instead of fixing things I was slowly throwing chairs off the Titanic.

Mother started railing at me as I got her to write a reduced amount to the phone company for a very overdue bill. I tried to turn her mood around. "We've been together for over a month and we had a really nice time. We had delicious meals together, read together, and I hope you can remember those good times. That's what I want to remember." I leaned over, kissed her check and told her I loved her.

"I don't know about that," she retorted, sharply.

I left the room to get my bags before Alex arrived to take me to the airport, telling myself, "That's not my mother talking, it's the disease." The South would not rise again. I was no longer in cahoots with denial.

From before Thanksgiving until MLK day Mother had been, except for a week, in her daughters' care. As Bev fumed, "Of course she did better with us. She was coddled, fed, entertained, and taken care of every minute." True, but I doubt she remembered it that way. She became incensed because I got her a TV that worked, color-coded all her meds, got her car a new battery, figured out why her phone didn't work, put the lock back in the doorknob, and found out that she was washing her clothes by spritzing Spray 'n Wash into the washing machine water. She saw my actions as invasive. To belabor a metaphor, like the planting of kudzu, we were a rescue operation gone wrong.

With the wisdom of hindsight I consider taking Mother back to Memphis my biggest mistake. I regret that in spite of all the signs, I followed her wishes. Occasionally I still torture myself with "if only." If only I had stopped the trajectory with a different decision. If only I had said to my soon-to-be-ex-boss, "I'm not coming back for my last two weeks of work." But I needed the salary in the face of financial uncertainties, and Judy would be in Memphis in ten days to take Mother to the doctor. Judy asked, as if prescient, "Can you imagine what can happen in ten days?" The worst did, much to our sorrow, come to pass.

On the plane home I read beautiful poems by Shawn Fawson about her mother's Alzheimer's, elegiac images of her mother being surrounded by snow. Fawon's poignant, lingering descriptions of a person disappearing into the whiteness reverberated through my tightly-wound nerves.

> *"To find her, I make myself a stranger, come to her like an open cage. But nothing I try touches her inside. Her life belongs to another story, the one where rain shudders to snow and covers every bend of the road as if in search of something. What does it matter now – she doesn't feel strange or cold. Why else does she wander barefoot into the storm if not to name what's left of our world before the next act of erasure?"*

All the unusual snow we'd experienced during the past few months gleamed like a physical expression of metaphysical depths. I thought of Mother's erasure. While my plane back to Seattle sat on the frigid Minneapolis tarmac awaiting some computer part, I reached for those good memories I had challenged Mother to retain. The minutes dragged on the runway, and I cradled a time when Mother and I shared food and blessings beneath white mountains, surrounded by loving family. Her observations about her youth, given in response to my inquiries as we passed the January dampness in Seattle, shimmered in my memory. She told me how I spit up on her new dress as a baby when she was on the way to her high school reunion, how Elois and Jack went one Saturday afternoon to get married, but it wasn't eloping. They had no wedding reception and no party, because there wasn't money for such things. Who would paint those pointillistic scenes when she was covered in the snow of Alzheimer's?

Back in Seattle Mother's impression tinted my house. I wanted to embrace her and tell her I loved her. I cursed modern medicine, some collection of current medications that extended longevity, but only a scarecrow remained, a husk in a field talking to the corn.

Mother called Bev, saying that it was lonesome since I left. *Mother did say that you had some rough spots,* Bev emailed. *That it's hard to have someone taking over your life. I said I just thought we were trying to help her. She said I guess I don't see it that way. OK, model daughter who's fallen off her pedestal, hero, saint, sleep well.*

I began to realize how distance muted Mother's problems. I talked to her several times a day, and except when she called to ask my sisters' birthdays, she almost convinced me she was on top of everything. Our shadows again partners in crime. But then it would slip out: a problem with another bill or another daily task flummoxing her. On the other hand, just when we'd write her off, she would see through our schemes with "I'm NOT stupid!"

An email from Bev: *Crazy! Thanks for checking up on all of these unpaid bills and accounts gone to the collection agency. I talked to Mother tonight, and those represent unfinished and unaccomplished tasks to her. So even though she isn't dealing with them herself, she feels the stress of something she can't handle. She said that she had talked to her neighbor Denise about driving her to appointments and to the store, but they hadn't come to any agreement. I'll call Denise this weekend. I was yelling and yelling to be heard.*

My "Lou Report" to Bev and Judy: *We need a contingency plan about the doctor. Judy is going to offer to take her to Chattanooga after her appointment with Dr. Powers, but after all the time away from home, it's going to be hard to get Mother to budge. She told me more than once that her traveling days are over. If (I hope, I hope) she does have all the tests run, there is a good possibility she could get a bad report. Maybe I'll need to go back and spend a week or two with her. We can't just leave her there alone.*

Mother was bilious in her assertions that she was fine and staying put in Memphis. Like Obama said at that time about the economy, we knew about Mother: it's going to get worse before it gets better. Judy firmly told her, "You're moving in February!" Having lost all sense of time, Mother readily agreed with Judy.

I bemoaned to anyone who would sympathize that I did not know what to do about Mother. Mother needed our assistance, desperately, but had a million illusions about why she was fine. (Say "fine" with a flat "i" and the contented Memphis accent, that lazy tongue of uncontested living.) A friend gave me the phone number of an elder consultant, someone her law firm recommended. Elder consultants are trained experts in dealing with such conundrums. When I talked to this consultant, she basically said we could not make Mother move or go into assisted living. She thought we had missed our "window" and drastic measures were going to be required. "If you miss the opportunity for moving them, they dig in their heels and it's hard make it happen." Just what I needed to hear; the window had closed, and we had missed the opportunity to move Mother, bemused and resigned, into assisted living in a daughter's zip code. She echoed my cousin's dire evaluation. We had waited too late.

I made a business trip from Seattle to eastern Washington on the last day of January. I was sick of airports, of lugging heavy bags down long, monotonous hallways, tired of cramming my coat into the overhead bins. I wanted a respite from traveling, to be at home where I could collect my wits and energy. Our collective sisterhood felt overwhelmed and exhausted. Like millions of Americans at that time the rigors of the Great Recession confined us. We struggled to pay our bills and manage our lives. Judy's husband Buddy had the unenviable position of being in the ranks of the early unemployed; manufacturing had been a leading indicator of bad times, and he had been a plant manager. That eastern Washington trip was my last duty before being downsized from my job. Still I found no excuses when I reconsidered how we mishandled Mother. I expected better from myself.

Chapter 12

MY PERSONAL SUMMONS TO MEMPHIS

"I wanted to get out of Mississippi in the worst way. Go back? What would I want to go back for?"

Muddy Waters

February 1, 2009

I reclined, splayed on my sofa, its purple fabric as dark as the ink imprinted on my hands from the (now defunct) Seattle P-I newspaper. The phone rang. I turned down the jazz on Sunday Side Up to hear Bev tell me that Mother had been taken to ER at the Memphis East Hospital with what looked like a stroke. Downplaying the event, all the participating friends, neighbors, and relatives around Mother said she seemed to be okay and she recognized them. Still, as legal power of everything, I needed to get to Memphis immediately.

Bev said, "I hope they at least keep Mother in the hospital overnight."

"Yeah," I agreed. "She's eighty-seven years old with high blood pressure. The ambulance ride alone might do her in."

Bev served as dispatcher during the morning crisis, due thankfully to her clandestine conversations with Mother's neighbors. From Memphis to California to Seattle to Chattanooga calls bounced to the medic, to Alex, calls with social security numbers, with a million questions. On the positive side, Mother would have all those tests she had resisted, and everyone would have to face what we had seen. Obviously, she could no longer live alone.

I asked Alex in one of many phone calls, "Was Mother glad to see you at ER?" I rushed around the house, collecting the trash and recycling the newspapers.

"I wouldn't say *that*."

The word "agitated" was used often.

This was not the medic's first visit to Mother. Another of her secrets. The medics knew her, Alex explained.

I paused, "I didn't know the medics had been there. The firemen for sure. Three times I think."

"Good to know your emergency providers," Alex deadpanned.

In less than three hours, I went from Sunday slug to sitting on a flight south. After a dozen family phone calls, I got a pricey airline ticket, gathered all the necessary legal papers, did a cursory house cleaning, showered, got my lovely neighbor Lil to take me to the airport, and arrived in time to stand, adrenaline still pumping, and wait in all the airport lines. Collapsed into the narrow airplane seat, my worst nightmare had materialized: Mother in a life-threatening situation and we, her daughters, reacting from afar.

I arrived in Memphis after midnight, and true to his good nature, Alex scooped me up at the airport and took me to Mother's home, reassuring me there was no reason to go the hospital at such a late hour. Drained, I concurred.

It was disconcerting to be in Mother's home without her. In the past her presence had emanated from her immaculate abode. That night when I turned on the lights, the rooms reflected a frantic state of mind: lamps on the floor, lined up against the wall as if awaiting a firing squad, lamp shades scattered like collateral damage; two blood pressure cuffs and batteries heaped beside her favorite chair. I walked through the condo picking up unplugged appliances and phones. A trail of her fecal-colored handprints mapped the hallway of her panic.

In the antique-filled guest bedroom I opened my suitcase, curious if I'd packed any pajamas. I found another pair of jeans, a couple of shirts, my toothbrush and a bevy of essential oils. I traveled with more essential oils than clothes.

When I got to ICU early the next morning, Judy was sitting in a chair reading "*The 36 Hour Day.*" She and her husband Buddy had arrived at the hospital in the middle of the night. Buddy went to his parents' house in Memphis, while Judy stayed with Mother in the ICU glass closet. Whispering, Judy and I shared details: Mother had suffered a brain infarct and a hemorrhagic stroke. No conclusions could be made about when either of those had happened, though from the CAT scan it appeared the bleeding had stopped. The nurses hurriedly took all my powers-of papers, and I began reading and signing hospital forms. Page after long page. Copies of the DNR were made.

Mother looked so frail, hooked up to a plethora of cords, covered by heart wires, stints and nose tubes. Digital numbers blinked on the monitors. She struggled to talk.

With garbled speech she directed, "Let's get me up." She fumbled with all the cords and IVs. Disoriented: another hospital understatement applied to Mother.

She looked at me with terrified eyes. I leaned close to her, touched her arm, and spoke tenderly into her ear, "Do you feel bad?"

She shook her head a feeble yes.

"Are you scared?"

Another slight nod yes, tears in her eyes.

If I thought this my worst nightmare, it quickly became apparent that it was certainly Mother's too. Her prayer that "the Lord will take me in my sleep at home" did not include the terror accosting her in the hospital.

Every communication trial was futile. "Do you know your name?" the nurse asked. Mother looked at her, perplexed. More questions and no connections. Then as the nurse left the ICU room, Judy told Mother that this, her night nurse, was leaving for the day. Somewhere, amid brain tangles and a blood blob, Mother found her lovely southern charm; she smiled at the nurse and spoke clearly. "Thank you, dear."

Next came the hospital battery of intrusive tests: EEG, EKG, echo gram, wires taped roughly to Mother's forehead, impatient tech staff scolding her not to move, all of it bewildering and irritating Mother. Tests scheduled for an hour stretched twice that long.

After that, Mother passed from a sweet, dazed phase into her "agitated" state. In a vocabulary of euphemisms, the word "agitated" reigned. It required Judy, Buddy and me to keep Mother in bed, while she keened, begged us to let her go and tried to pull out her tubes. In vain I asked the nurse for more meds. So the three of us, son-in-law and daughters, stood around the hospital bed reaching across its raised side rails, and softly held Mother's arms and legs to protect her from getting up and falling, or from something worse. We sang to her, a hymnal full of the songs of her life. Judy and Buddy, dedicated Christians, were a ready repository for the verses that eluded me. "I Come to the Garden Alone," "This Little Light of Mine," "What a Friend We Have in Jesus," "How Great Thou Art." My voice cracked with the emotion of that heritage and for my disturbed mother. The songs soothed Mother, but merely temporarily. Stranded in the alien space of the ICU windowed room, Mother screamed like a banshee and wrestled against us. We sang, only a few feet from the central nurses' station. No one came to help. Then, as Mother continued to flail, a nurse arrived, saying, "We're moving her out of ICU." Stunned, we offered to accompany Mother, but the nurses were deluded and sent us ahead, thinking they could handle her. When they finally arrived to ICU Step Down, the nurses admitted Mother had outlasted them with her tenacity and fear.

Walking across the sidewalk between the hospital lobby and parking garage to attend to some errand, I called Seattle and cancelled the two weeks of work I had scheduled. I could see that I was going to be in Memphis longer than my two pair of jeans had anticipated.

The hospital days passed in dog years, Judy and Buddy went back to Chattanooga, and Mother began the hallucinations. I held her hand one minute, as she affectionately touched my face and smoothed my hair; then off into la-la land, where, bless her heart, she acted slightly goofy, certain she was working at Kennedy Hospital in the quartermaster department during World War II where something was missing. "We don't know what happened to it. Twenty-five pounds short. Somebody is going to get in trouble," she worried, unaware of her skimpy washed-out green hospital gown. She indicated for me to move things on the wall, though in reality nothing was there. I pretended, she watched my movements, disagreeing or nodding her head, orchestrating with her hands bruised from all the IVs. Finally she acknowledged I had fixed some sight bothering only her.

In the afternoon Mother cooed, "You're so pretty." That night she asked for a knife or fork or file to get away from there. Mother's forays into the nether became more insistent, "I've got to get out there, he wants to know the price of silver, she wants jewelry." She would shriek, "Why can't you just let me go. I've had a good life." The contest to leave the hospital would escalate. One day it took almost five hours, and she landed a solid slap on my face. It required me, three nurses, two injections, Uncle Bill and Aunt Donna Jean, Tanya the night nurse, restraints, another injection, my panicked call to the doctor, yet another injection, Uncle Bill, Aunt Donna Jean and me with Mother <u>in restraints</u> to keep her in bed. The staff handled Mother's taunts politely, apologetic about the restraints. I hated having to make that decision. My hippocampus cemented that awful sight into stone: my mother, hands and feet tightened to the bed in restraints, fighting against family and staff, uncontrollable after powerful sedatives. She chaffed against the restraints, which, of course, were charged on her hospital bill. The nurses put the meds in her IV, I spoke softly to her, but Mother spewed rancor. I went into the hospital hall and sobbed.

Passing people cautiously asked, "Are you all right? Can we get you anything?"

"Not really," and I thanked them, gulping big sobs.

The next night during my nap, mother succeeded in her great escape and landed on the floor, bloody injuries where the IVs were ripped out, flimsy gown caught in a jumble of wires. Ever the unrelenting caretaker Mother had attempted to get a roast out of the oven during her hallucinations. The loud alarms of her disconnected wires woke me and I found her naked, on her knees beside the bed. I put my arms around my terrified mother, until the nurses came running into the room.

Bev entered the sister exchange, California for Chattanooga. However, by the time Bev got to Memphis, Mother lay unresponsive. The nurses suggested it was all the meds Mother had been given to stop her warfare. Bev's introduction into hospital pain came when Mother groaned fitfully, "Take me home, Bev-er-leee, get me out of here! Take me home, Howard!" Just when we accepted Mother's turn for the worst, she perked up, reaching like a little bird for a kiss on the lips. Bev grinned. "She came out to play with me."

Bev entertained Mother with photos, asking, "Who's this? Who's that?"

Finally Bev pointed to Mother in one of the snapshots, joking, "Who's this?"

"Yours truly!" Mother grinned.

"We should remember these minutes" Mother declared. From the way she hesitated Mother was probably looking for a word other than "minute." Although the truth of those days was measured in small, cherished moments.

"This is your doctor," we reminded Mother as another white jacket dashed into the room.

She fixed a polite smile. "You're a doctor now?"

Too many times to count we heard from doctors, "a stroke exacerbates Alzheimer's." This anguish had Mother's blood pressure off the charts. She had a nitrogen patch to lower her hypertension, but it wasn't working. Jack, the handsome young nurse from Kenya who spoke four languages in calm, accented tones, explained the nitrogen patch to me. I wondered to myself, "How do you say vascular dilator in Kikuyu?"

The doctor train chugged along, and we asked daily for a prognosis. A waiting game, they warned, maybe months to see if the stroke damage was permanent. We torpedoed direct queries at the doctors who brushed into mother's room and out in an instant. The neuro guy had bad breath, which sullied the air like the news he delivered: Mother had to go into long-term nursing care this week and she was too sick to move out of town. I sobbed when he left the room; our worst fears a reality. My apologies to Dylan "but I was stuck inside of Memphis with the Mother blues again." The internist, yesterday's rudest doctor, oozed sucrose after learning that our cousin was head of ER. "I'll pray for you," he proffered in lieu of answers. When he demurred to further questions with a forced smile, "that's a brake question. I'm the transmission guy," I found his analogy disparaging to Daddy's business. The heart doc, a nice young man whom Mother had dumped as her physician, shook his head unsurprised. On Mother's office chart he had noted that her hypertension made her a high risk for stroke. Dr. Powers, the gerontologist Mother had seen only once, did not have visitation privileges at Memphis East; he told Judy on the phone, "Ten days in the hospital to stabilize her, then an ambulance to Chattanooga."

Due to Medicare payment limits, the effort had already begun to move Mother into a rehab facility. Finding a rehab facility, however, was like some disappointing sorority rush where rejections needed no explainations. "She's not Sigma Sigma material," we intoned in our high school sorority smugness. Maybe critical care facilities had the same ambiguous standards. In order to get Mother into rehab, the hospital scheduled her for physical therapy (lower body), occupational therapy (life skills and small motor), and speech therapy. Mother needed to show progress with these therapists for a facility to accept her. Medicare paid 100% for 20 days then 80% for a total of three months of rehab, as long as Mother improved.

The speech therapist was a dream come true. She answered our questions, explaining what happened during Mother's left-hemisphere brain hemorrhage, how it affected her speech patterns, and how we could help Mother relearn to talk. We loved that speech therapist, Mary Catherine, a sweet woman who brightened our dismal hospital days.

"It's like all the brain's information is kept in a card file," Mary Catherine described. "And with a stroke that file is dumped out on the floor. When your mother is asked a question, her brain reaches into that pile of messed-up cards on the floor and pulls a card. It may or may not be the right one. Sometimes there's no card to be found. Eventually, with therapy and healing, some of that card file can be put back together. But usually it's not exactly like it was. Often some cards, information or memories, are never retrieved."

I pictured random cards, language skills, names and faces, scattered beneath her brain's AD damage. Digging through the tangled mess in Mother's brain made finding those strewn brain cards as elusive as tadpoles in a pond murky with mud and algae.

Mary Catherine also explained the brain's automatics. These were verbal expressions, spoken so often in life, so automatically, that they existed beyond the disheveled card file. "Everyone has automatics," Mary Catherine said, "but not all of those automatics are as nice as your Mother's." Mother could still plainly say many things we'd heard from her our entire lives. "Well, I tell ya," she'd allow, followed by mangled syllables. When we left the room, with nary a slur, she'd ask, "Do ya need anything?"

Mary Catherine had flash cards with words and pictures for Mother to identify. Mother tried hard, using phonetics to pronounce those words. Sounding out each syllable, Mother spoke the word correctly, without any idea what those clear enunciations meant, the meaning not to be found in her chaotic card file. Those phonetics were the automatics of a sterling student eighty years later, ever the precocious daughter of an angular school principal. "I've never seen anyone else do that!" Mary Catherine said admiringly.

Mary Catherine would show Mother a picture. Instead of admitting she didn't know what it was, Mother would clutch the card to her chest, exclaiming, "That's soooo adorable!" That gesture became an integral part of Mother's physical vocabulary. When we showed her a photo of her great-grand daughter, Mother hugged the photo with "isn't that cute!" Mother's inarticulate vowels and consonants were expressed by shrugging her shoulders and age-spotted arms in major consternation, her bodily "I don't know."

Bev and I created our own occupational therapy. We had Mother folding bath cloths that we brought from her home closet, reading get-well cards, which she eventually tore in half, and working large puzzles. It was frustrating to Mother at times, those questions she couldn't answer. "Let's don't mess with that now," she'd say. To the relentless question of "do you know where you are?" Mother would admit, "a lot of this doesn't add up." One day Mother couldn't take it any longer. When Mary Catherine posed some familiar question, Mother vented, "It's all bull shit." Our Sunday School teaching, morality-preaching Mother finally came out with an automatic we had never heard her say. Then she paused, "Bird shit!" As if "bull" was the bad word. It was "sooo adorable."

Mother was public property, suffering the indignities of dementia. The present was lost to her, caught in the brier patch of her brain; otherwise, she would have been horrified about the exposure of her tracing-paper skin and bare bottom for the parade of gentle strangers who bathed her sagging body.

We took turns staying with Mother at night, sleeping in our clothes on the narrow sofa, covered by a white cotton blanket. The darkness of the hospital room was round like a well. Just as fitful sleep slipped through the thick night, the heavy room door opened, then light from the sterile hallway folded into a trapezoid on the floor. The nurse's aid flicked on the overhead fixture and pushed in a noisy cart with medical paraphernalia. Covering my eyes for a moment, I willed myself into conviviality from my suspension in a fog of sleep crystals. I silently blessed these people for their attentions to my mother, for never flinching about the diarrhea, the blood or the smells. In those long hours I had learned the stories of those who tended my mother: about their grandchildren, about a wife who was a preacher, about the bank job lost in the recession. It was Memphis, the first decade of the twenty-first century, and many of these caretakers were black.

The strong attendant and I lifted Mother to the edge of the hospital bed. She looked at his African-American face in panic, "Don't kill me! Please don't kill me! I don't have any money! Don't kill me! I don't have a dime!"

Quickly, I tried to deflate her embarrassing pleas with "no, of course you don't have any money because we're taking care of you."

Startled she grasped she was empty-handed, "Where's my purse? Where are my rings? Who took them?" She turned her head toward the stoic black man carefully taking her blood pressure.

The next day Mother assessed her intruders, "These nigras," she said, alluding to the black men who gingerly changed her diapers, "I love them." Then she paused, reconsidering from the static of her short-circuited memories, "Well, not really."

The whiplash of Mother's condition led us to believe that she might be dying; while she did have times of clarity, mostly she weakened. In the face of this decline, Judy and Buddy brought their young adult offspring to tell their grandmother good-bye. Mother with her limited speech managed to talk to each of those grandkids, wanting as ever to know about their lives. We got Mother out of the hospital bed and sat her in a chair. She smiled for the family paparazzi, holding hands and kissing her grandkids. While Mother napped and the guys stayed with her, we women went back to the condo to sort through boxes laden with bank statements and mail, and to throw away canned goods years out-of-date.

My sisters and I went out to dinner to talk realistically about what might be ahead. We attempted to make plans for Mother's future care, with a bare minimum of information. Hindering Mother from a nursing facility were her continually spiking blood pressure and her aberrant behavior. We all agreed that I would stay with Mother in Memphis for as long as it took.

After that night in a real bed at Mother's home, I returned to the hospital room to find Bev and Judy clustered around the white dry-erase board with our favorite nurse. We trusted the nurses, recognizing that the lower on the hospital food chain, the more obliging. We wanted to clarify Mother's array of meds, with meticulous explanations from our trusted nurses. I watched, with pride, as my two sisters wrote with blue felt pens the names of psychotropic meds, along with indications and hours of administration, accompanied by blood pressure numbers and other vitals. Besides blood pressure meds, in times of stress Mother could be given Ativan as a sedative, and Haldol and Abilify as anti-psychotic drugs, prescribed by the psychiatrist in the classic suits and high heels. No doctor conveyed the risks of giving Mother those meds. Maybe the Haldol did work for a while, or maybe it was all chance. Once I was confident giving Mother foot massages had settled her down, but the next time I tried it and she couldn't kick me enough with those size eleven feet of hers.

Mother, still unhinged, was moved to the neuro floor. The Doc train grew, adding a passenger car with social workers to help with "where next?" It did take a village and a long choo-choo of experts to deal with the decisions and paperwork.

On good days the ladies from the church filed into Mother's hospital room, wearing their blazers, necklaces, and fancy scarves. They held hands with my mom for a few minutes until she begged them to take her home, and they left the room with a story and tears. Familiar faces peeked around the thick hospital door: neighbors from the columned house, Walls relatives, my chaplain friend Linda with her two generations of red-headed progeny, and church deacons. They brought homemade brownies, banana bread, big baskets of snacks, crossword puzzles, and best of all, memories.

Mary, a church friend of sixty years and now a white-haired energy ball built like a short running back, bounded into the hospital room enthusiastically. She had peach pickin' stories. Another church lady added: "I was done in 30 minutes, but Mary and Lou were still looking around for the biggest and best peaches. Mary had a picker utensil and Lou would follow her around with 'where did you get those nice peaches?'"

All the women needed to talk of their alarm over Mother's decline, either to complete the story or to allay their own guilt.

"I told her she needed to go to the doctor," one assured me, dabbing at her wet eyes.

"Preachin' to the choir" became my standard reply.

"I didn't know what to do," another bemoaned.

Neither did we, I wanted to shout. Instead I simply nodded in sympathy.

Alton Wayne, one of Daddy's brothers, spoke of Mother's tempering influence on the Walls family. "After the war all the brothers were drinking and going out to clubs. Then Howard married Lou. She had a lot to do with changing that." In the telling he expressed respect for her effect as the moral compass. Mother had obviously not said "bird shit" around Alton Wayne.

Bev admitted, "But Mother was really uncomfortable at first because the Walls were so well dressed and good looking."

"Well, she was nervous," Alton agreed in his slow, methodical speech.

The literal 24/7 at the hospital alternated among our sisterhood. I needed to go to the bank to figure out Mother's finances. As I left, Mother chirped from her hospital bed, "Be careful. Can I get ya anything?"

"No thanks, I'm fine." I smiled, buttoning my coat.

With an automatic she saved specifically for me, her unruly daughter, she added, "Behave yourself!"

The mailboxes at the Magnolia Condominium Village were centrally located. All of Mother's neighbors talked about her walking to the mailboxes and enjoying that meeting place. Surely, as her short-term memory eroded, she made that trek to the mailboxes many times a day. Between the hospital and bank, I stopped for Mother's mail and saw her postman. I explained to him about being Miz Lou's daughter and that she was in the hospital.

"Oh, she told me about you and your sisters when she went to visit you over the holidays." He stuffed more mail into the slots. "She said y'all wanted her to move out there, but she said she wasn't gonna do it. Not ever."

I had to chuckle. Even the African-American postman knew she was not going to move, but her deluded daughters never gave up the dream.

My life was measured that February by the five miles driven in my mother's old car between the hospital and her home, trading hospital shifts with whichever sister was in Memphis. In that straight shot in the ancient gas-burning car I listened to NPR, feigning normalcy, wishing that classical music could appease the demons transferred from Mother's brain to my emotions. Like her, my nights and days were reversed, and doctors sucked. Entering Mother's hospital room, I immediately gave Bev the keys and some verbal GPS of where to find the car. "Second floor, third row, on the left-hand side, about half way down."

We were subsumed in hospital ennui: acutely aware of the lonely walk down the sanitized hallways, the window away from other rooms with the best cell phone reception and the "4" button on the elevator that didn't light. Long-timers like ourselves stood out. We might be wearing "house shoes" and we usually carried a large bag with extra clothes, personal diversions, and objects from home for the patient. Slightly dragging, we did not move with the hope of the fresh visitors bringing balloons and flowers. The consternation on our faces could have been about recent test results or wondering where we parked our cars.

Mother continued her attempts to manipulate us away from the bed so that she could flee. "Now y'all go on home," she suggested kindly. "Go out and have fun." She threw off covers and sheets blocking her way, "Put on y'all's pajamas and go to bed." Mother sunk deeper into her nighttime deliriums. As she called by name all those who had gone ahead to the Promised Land without her, I transversed my childhood, recognizing that the people and life Mother loved had disappeared. I fell asleep only to be jolted awake by a blur of her naked flesh on the floor again. The nurse reassured me, "You have to sleep." Mother whimpered, pestering with her IV lines for hours. Her forays into "psychosis" escalated, and she spent bleak nights in her ghost town. She was put on Seroquel, an anti-schizophrenia drug.

We took precarious walks on the emotional edge with Mother. We dallied in her long-gone world, pretending for her, "Howard's at work." "Just kill me!" she cadged. There was no turning back, not enough Haldol or Ativan. She ranted, prayed, kicked and hated us in those crazy hours.

After long days and nights of hallucinatory torment she spent all her strength. A slight touch on her shoulder deterred forward momentum, but she didn't quit demanding to talk to the sheriff or police or "head head nurse" or president of this bank. "Don't do me this way!" she'd plead. The shit and blood everywhere seemed etched into our vision, but in truth the horrors were masked by Mother's lifetime of determination and her ceaseless patience with her grandchildren.

She no longer connected with her swipes and instead bent back my fingers when I held her hands to keep her in bed. "Let me up!" she demanded. "I've got to get back to my dorm room. You are a vicious, vicious woman. The most vicious woman I've ever seen." She tried a different ploy. "I'll give you $5 to get me out of here." The next day we kidded that Cassandra, the lively Physical Therapist, earned that five-dollar bribe by getting Mother up on the walker.

In that southern state of institutionalized religion I was prayed over often and oratorically. In the middle of one dark night a chaplain came in. We stood in the hospital room without lights. Mother moaned.

"Can you imagine how lonely and frightening it is for someone in the hospital by themselves? It's a reflection on your mother that you're here with her now," he comforted me. I agreed tremulously, too tearful to admit that my mama had raised me right.

I had my own prayers, but kept getting more of the same: changing the diarrhea diapers of a mother who no longer knew me. Although I did think she recognized me when she demanded, "Get some decent clothes!"

Mother pleaded to get out of bed. We told her, "The doctors say no." But before we could finish she swept us aside, "That's immaterial."

We were encouraged when Mother fed herself, maneuvered precariously down the hospital corridors with a walker, and conversed with visitors. In her halting speech, Mother held forth, "It's nice to be nice to all. Meeting all these new people. If not tomorrow, the next day. New church, new experiences." And my favorite, "we did everything for love." Mother's sermons, Mother's prayers, Mother's life.

No wonder Mother wanted to get out of there, to return to an earlier innocence. Some afternoons Mother spouted from her Mississippi fever dreams, "Let's all move to Mississippi together. We don't see each other enough. And we live so close." Mississippi, that backward life she had sought to evade with the same vengeance she tried to hop over her hospital bed railings. Mississippi, more than an idyllic reminiscence, glowed as tomorrow's haven. Voices from her past, gliding like wraiths through the pastures of vermillion clover in Mississippi, beckoned her at night. She longed to follow them, into that carefree refrain. Or perhaps it was God she heard, calling her home.

Mother shared intimate afternoons with each of her daughters those weeks in the hospital. Bev brushed Mother's hair, and Judy read the Bible to her. Bev, catering to Mother's taste buds, brought her banana pudding and pork barbeque, the Holy Grail of southern cuisine. Mother ate heartily, with Bev's assistance. Daily I patted rose cream onto her cheeks and rubbed her forehead with essential oils. All the nurses commented on Mother's beautiful skin.

The pressure increased about finding Mother a rehab facility. We took Mother off IV fluids, off the nitro patch, and off anything holding her in hospital hell. She had been there almost three weeks. Bev booked her necessary flight back to California: she had a husband, daughter and job to attend. I looked at a nursing facility that had an empty bed. It was awful, elders asleep in wheelchairs in the dreary hallways. I looked at another that was excellent with no available space.

Another brain scan revealed nothing to explain Mother's decline: no TIAs, no more strokes, and the brain bleed appeared to be shrinking. We had to get her to a rehab facility.

Our dearth of choices discouraged us. However, at Kenwood Mother could have a private room and the staff seemed caring. I read and signed all the papers to admit Mother there and wrote another check.

After being informed about the Memphis law that family could not spend the night at the nursing home, Bev interviewed several agencies that provided at-home, or in this case at-facility care; signed more papers; wrote another check and hired someone for a 12-hour shift at night. Between the angel-of-the-night and her daughters, Mother still had 24/7 care.

Another law prevented nursing facilities from giving psychotropic drugs to their patients. The Physician's Assistant expressed shock that the hospital had given them to Mother. We would have to see how her night went without those meds.

I went ahead to the nursing facility, while Bev rode over in the ambulance with Mother, who had lost all inhibitions and flashed the medics. As the stretcher moved her down the hall, Mother asked me, "Did we go to Tupelo?" Tupelo, Mississippi was where Aint E had been in the nursing facility. Shirley, an empathetic African-American woman, arrived for the night shift. Mother, a big smile on her shrinking face, eagerly hugged Shirley, convincing me that Mother thought she was in Tupelo, where she had admired the African-American women who had cared for Elois. Satisfied with Mother's safety and her imaginary return to Mississippi, Bev and I went back to the Mother's condo, the first night we had been there together in a very long time.

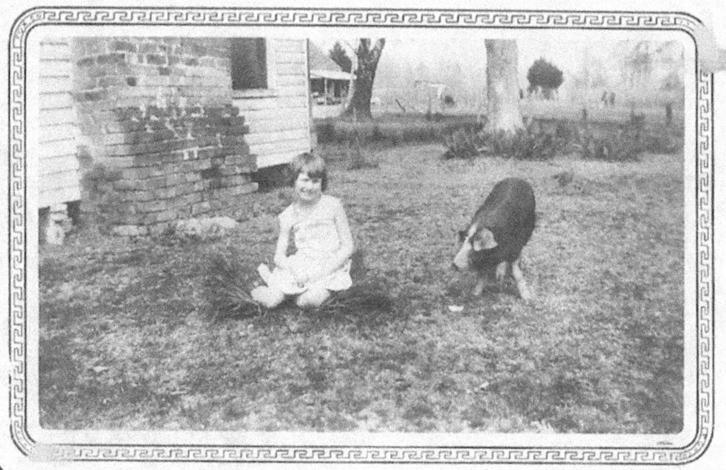

Willie Lou and her pet pig.

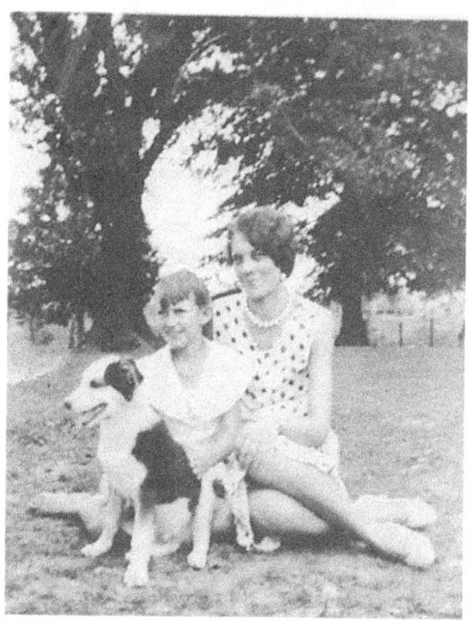

Mother with her dog Charlie and her cousin Gladys. Mother and Elois lived with Gladys in Memphis when they worked at Kennedy Hospital during World War II.

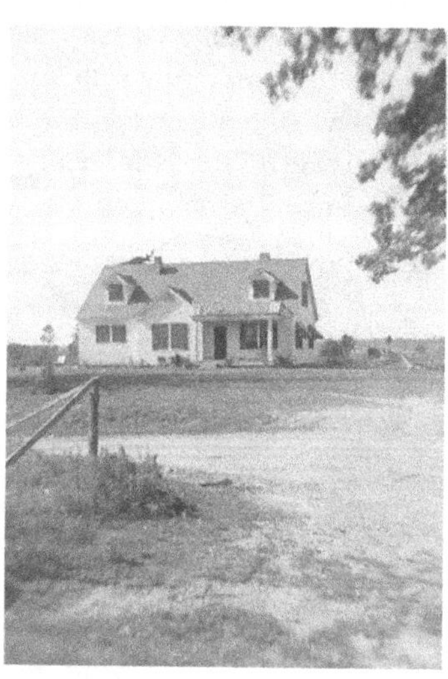

The Vinson house in Ellistown, Mississippi, built in the 1930s.

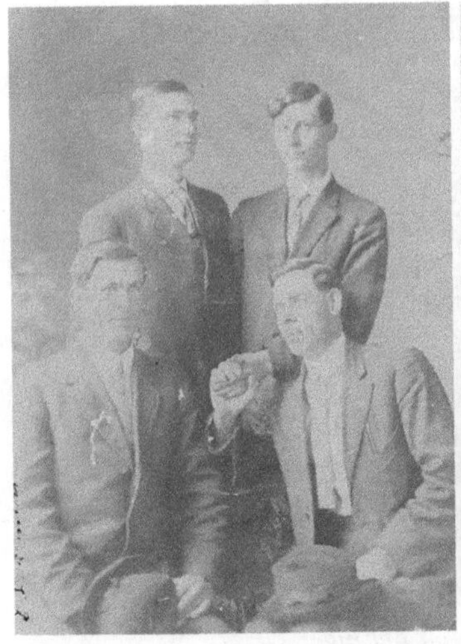

Papa Vinson and his uncles, the Robbins boys. Papa Vinson grew up in the same house with his uncles after his father died. I love that one of his uncles is holding Papa Vinson's hand.

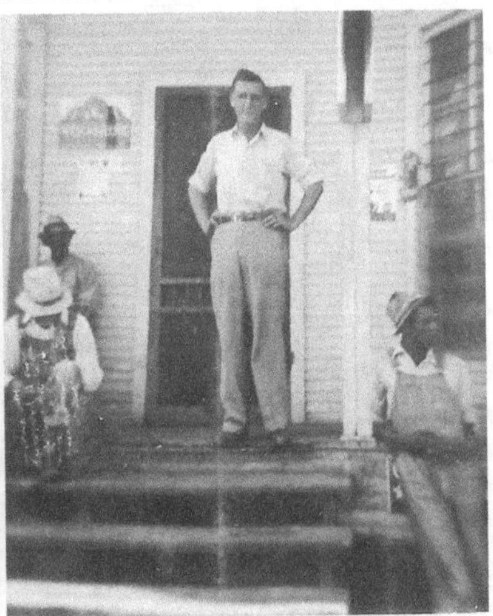

Papa Vinson at his store in Blair, Mississippi in the 1930s.

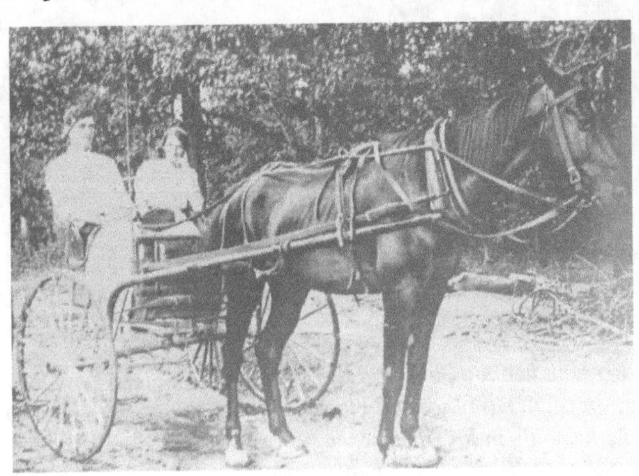

Papa Vinson and Mama Mat courting.

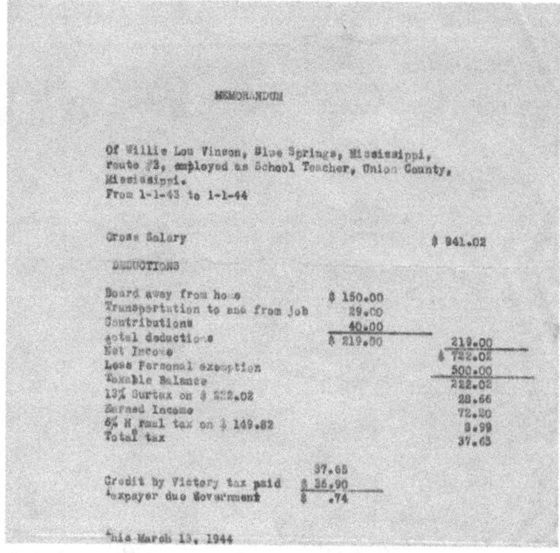

MEMORANDUM

Of Willie Lou Vinson, Blue Springs, Mississippi, route #3, employed as School Teacher, Union County, Mississippi.
From 1-1-43 to 1-1-44

Gross Salary		$ 941.02
DEDUCTIONS		
Board away from home	$ 150.00	
Transportation to and from job	29.00	
Contributions	40.00	
Total deductions	$ 219.00	219.00
Net Income		$ 722.02
Less Personal exemption		500.00
Taxable Balance		222.02
13% Surtax on $ 222.02		28.66
Earned Income		72.20
6% Normal tax on $ 149.82		8.99
Total tax		37.65
	37.65	
Credit by Victory tax paid	$ 36.90	
Taxpayer due Government	$ .74	

This March 13, 1944

Mother made $941 for teaching an entire year in the Delta. After expenses, she earned $722.

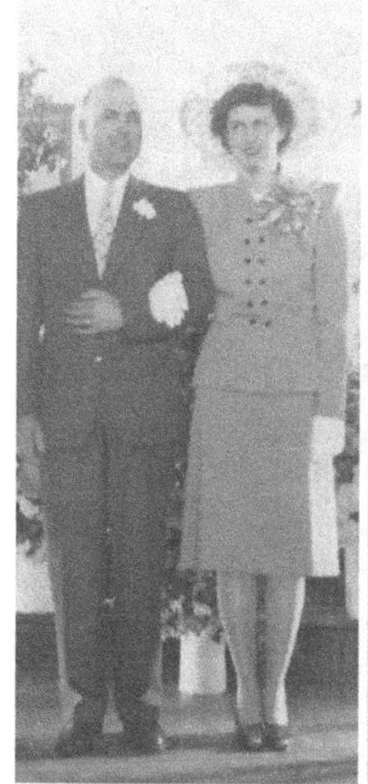

My parents were married at Ellistown Baptist Church in1946.

My dear Howard,

How strange it seems to be away from you so long. According to the theory of most people, one week, less than a week, isn't very long, but for me to be away from you who is close to me, who almost thinks for me and knows my every change of mind, is like an eternity. Truly to know, darling, that every day held no more than the days passed, no you, no dreaming, planning, doing and laughing, I don't think it would be worth the effort. To miss you is saying only words. But, honey, to know the longing in my heart to look and see you near-by would be knowing half the pain. I've wished for you so many times. Dot and I play a little game. Yesterday I said that you were coming last night. Today she asked if you came. Yes I said that it was late when you got here. On we go.

One of Mother's love letters to Daddy from 1946. Letters to him were saved in a box labeled "Howard." What a lovely surprise to find them!

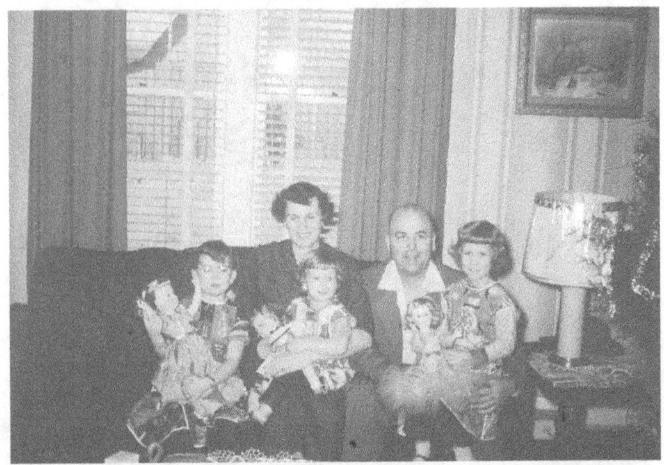

Christmas at Mama Mat and Papa Vinson's house in Blue Springs Mississippi. Me, Mother, Daddy, Judy and Bev. Our homemade aprons and dolls were presents.

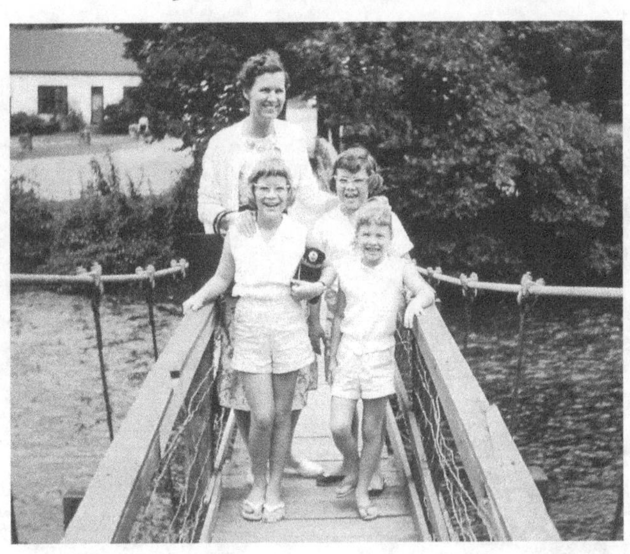

Mother, Beverly, me and Judy on a vacation in the Smoky Mountains.

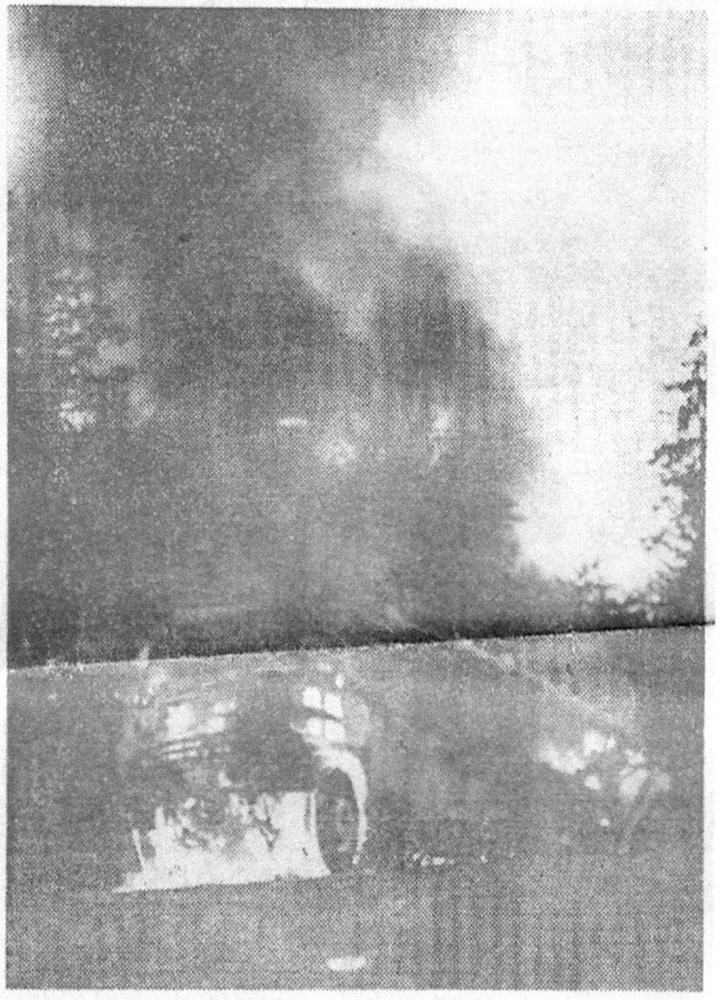

BLAZING BUS—At Newfound Gap, high in the mountain pass through Great Smoky Mountains National Park, the chartered bus carrying the Memphians flamed and exploded. They had stopped here to pray and admire the scene Thursday evening on their way home.

From the Commercial Appeal Newspaper, July 25, 1952. Mother saved the creased and tattered newspaper articles for over 60 years.

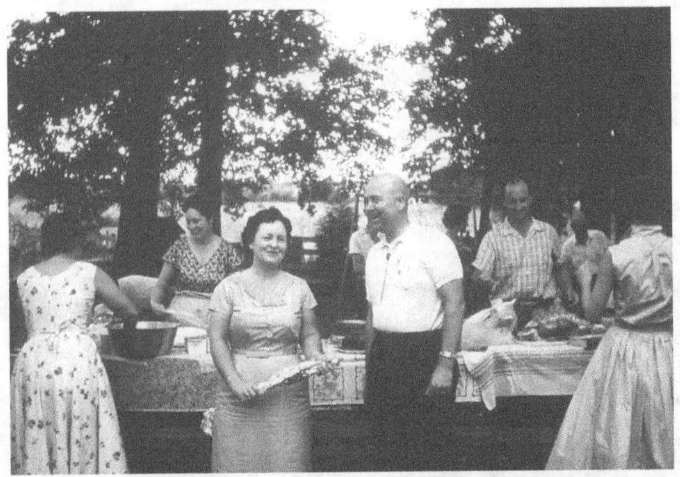

Daddy, center, at a Walls reunion in Mississippi.

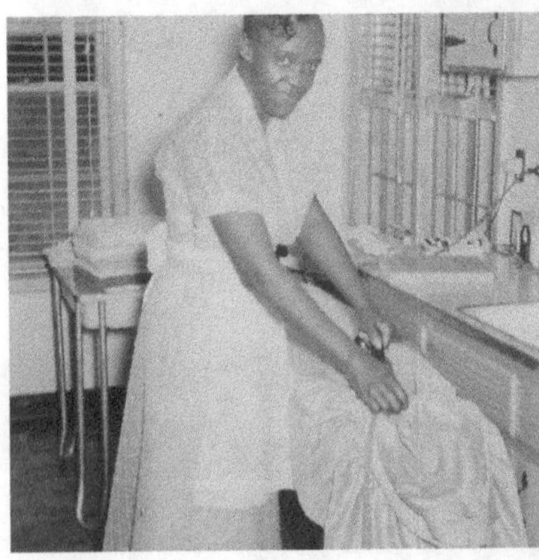

Nonie, our maid, in Memphis in the 1950s. She would be ironing when we got home from school, and she would stop ironing and pamper us with snacks and attention.

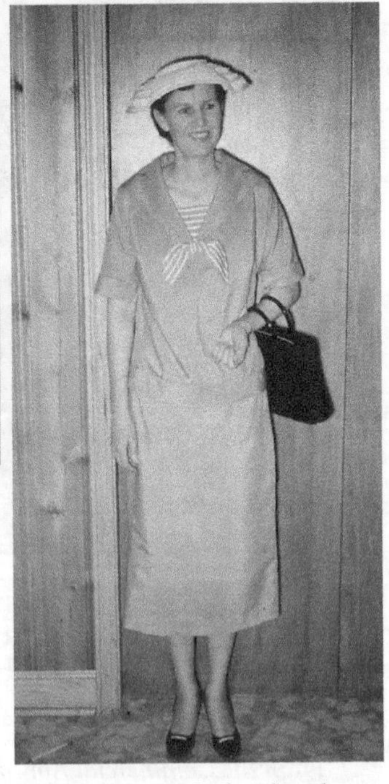

Mother ready for church.

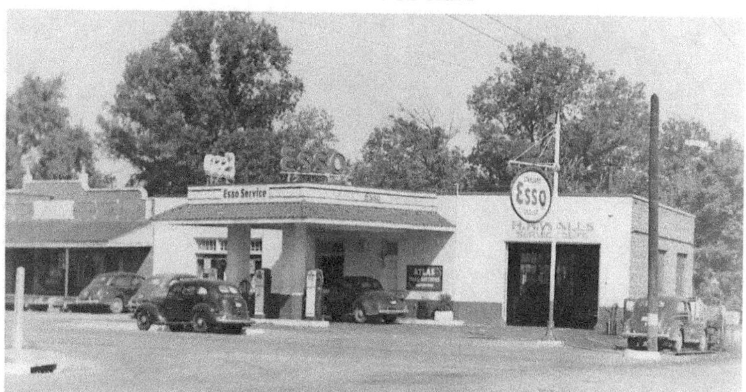

The original Esso station, 1940s, on the corner of Highland and Southern in Memphis. Daddy later bought the ice house next door to expand his business.

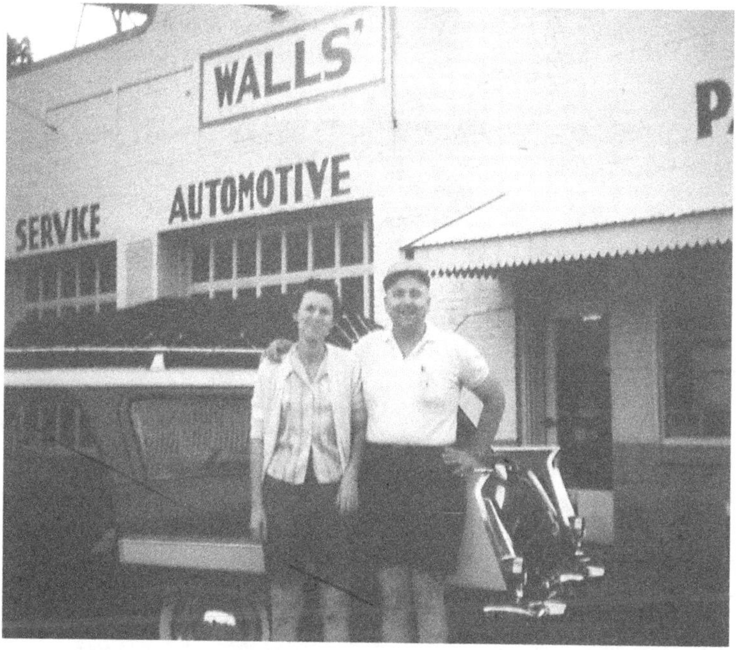

Daddy and Mother, ready for a family camping vacation to the West Coast,1950s.

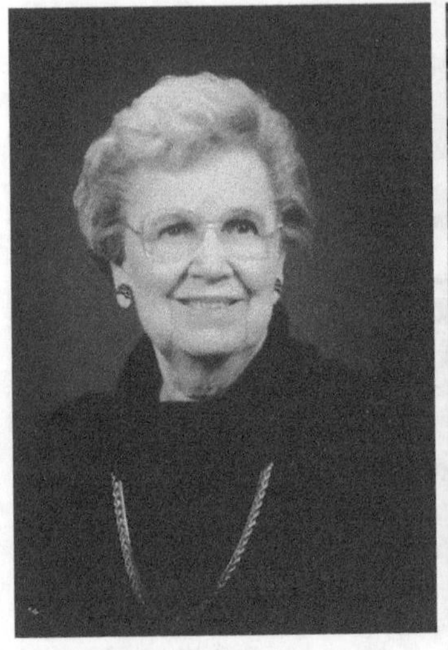

My beautiful and gracious Mother.

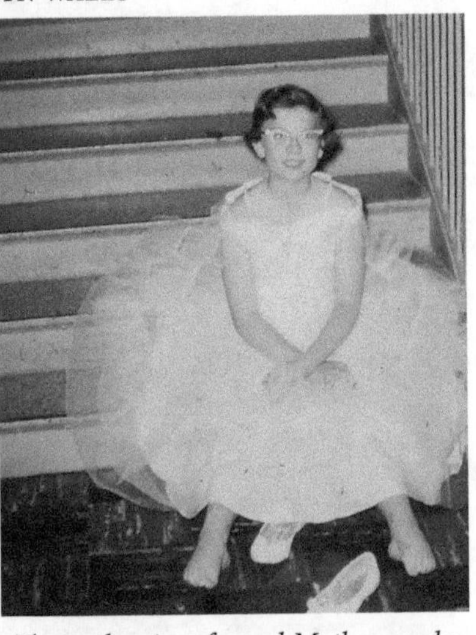

The author in a formal Mother made. Mother was an exquisite artist at creating our clothes.

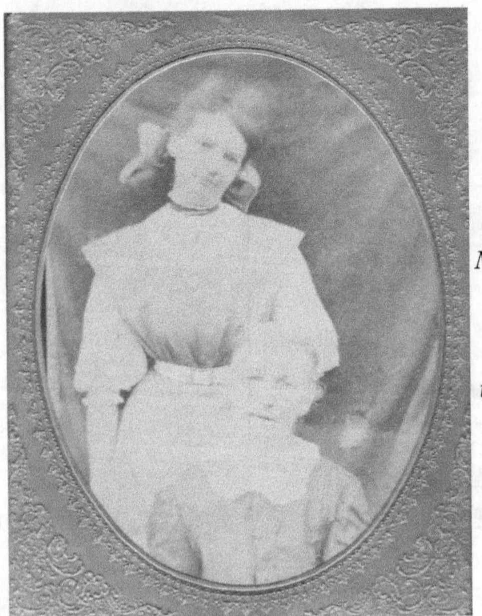

Granny Susie (sitting), Mother's grandmother, and Mama Mat (standing), my grandmother. This is the photo Mother mailed to me that I received after her death.

Chapter 13

A SCIENTIFIC AND A HOLISTIC VIEW FROM THE HOSPITAL

"Primum non nocere, (first, do no harm)."

Hippocratic oath

STROKES AND HEART DISEASE

In the hospital Mother was treated for a stroke and a brain bleed. Every forty seconds in the U.S. someone has a stroke, and in case anyone thinks a stroke is just something that happens to your grandmother, the incidence is rising among younger adults.[1]

A stroke is like the brain having a heart attack, and there are two different kinds. Eighty-seven percent are ischemic strokes, a result of obstruction in the blood vessels supplying the brain.[2] Atherosclerosis (those fatty or plaque deposits blocking blood flow) can happen in the brain just like to the heart.

Thirteen percent of strokes are hemorrhagic stroke,[3] also called a brain bleed, when a weakened vessel bursts and bleeds into the surrounding brain. One cause of weakened vessels can be consistent hypertension, which puts pressure on the brain. Either kind of stroke can damage the brain or kill the person. Mother, not content to be in only the top 87% with an ischemic stroke, also scored with the minority 13% by having a hemorrhagic stroke. Shockingly, she survived both. When I would say, "My mother had a stroke," folks would ask who found her. I explained, marveling at her toughness, "She never went down." She walked around outside looking for her long-dead husband, keys in her hands and plans to drive somewhere. Only she couldn't get the garage door to open. Her neighbors called 911.

Though too late for Mother, the nutritionist in me can't leave the topic of cardiovascular disease (CVD) without a few suggestions. As with every condition, we're stuck with our genetics. However, outside of that, decreasing stroke risk is immensely affected by lifestyle. Medical science has learned how to lower the risks of CDV: manage diabetes and high blood pressure; eat healthy; and <u>eliminate</u> tobacco and physical inactivity (*couchous potatoitis*).

Poor diet choices have long been implicated in poor heart health outcomes. According to the Center for Disease Control (CDC), over a million people die annually in the U.S. from diseases that are preventable and 80% of those preventable diseases result from food choices. "It is likely that a healthy diet has an effect on cardiovascular risk factors and cardiovascular disease, and that this is an important mechanism for reducing the risk of cognitive declines."[4] Those food deputies are getting the recognition they deserve! A study from Harvard cites the benefits of a plant-based diet. A plant-based diet low in animal fats is associated with a 20% decreased risk of type 2 diabetes; a healthy version of a plant-based diet reduced the risk of diabetes by 34%; but a less healthy version, I'm looking at you refined grains, potatoes and sugar-sweetened drinks, increased the risk by 16%.[5]

Mother would call me a broken record, but here's one more lecture about diet. Cut down on red and processed meats, including that all-time favorite, bacon. Just two slices of bacon a day can increase the risk of diabetes by more than 50%.[6] A 2012 study from Harvard verifies this risk: "Our study adds more evidence to the health risks of eating high amounts of red meat, which has been associated with type 2 diabetes, coronary heart disease and stroke." By substituting one serving of meat a day with poultry, fish, nuts, legumes or whole grains, risk of dying prematurely from CDV is reduced by 7-19%.[7]

There's more! Dump the margarine; say good-bye to as much processed food as possible; eat more fish, but not fried; eat more vegetables, more salads but with less salad dressing, and snack on fruits. Whole grains can lower your blood pressure: in one study three servings of whole grains daily for three months lowered systolic blood pressure by eight points.[8]

Low vitamin D impacts heart health. Low D levels increased the risk of stroke, stroke severity and fatality.[9] After a cardiac arrest, low D greatly increased the risk of poor neurological function.[10] Need more reasons for vitamin D awareness? Vitamin D may reduce plaque formation and blood pressure for patients with type 2 diabetes,[11] as well as diminish the risk of depression in stroke patients.[12] Studies continue to establish that results are "dose dependent," which means lower measures of vitamin D offered no improvement, while larger doses did make a difference.

Almost anyone can be deficient in vitamin D, no matter the weather. Deterrents to synthesizing D from sun include higher latitudes, air quality conditions, sunscreen, age, weight and darker skin pigmentation. The best answer to the question of how much vitamin D to take is with a 25-hydroxy vitamin D blood test.

Let's hear it for exercise one more time! A study completed in 2013 followed over 48,000 participants for six years and substantiated brisk walking, compared to running, as an effective means of lowering blood pressure.[13] Even small amounts of light-to-moderate exercise are beneficial for improved heart health.[14]

MEDICATIONS

Besides Mother's immediate danger from her stroked out brain and high blood pressure, the other major concern was her agitation, that euphemism for her uncontrollable behavior. She was dosed with anti-psychotic drugs, which we were told would address her relentless hours of hallucinations. Of course we were not experts on pharmaceuticals, and no one driving Mother's doctor locomotive told us the downsides of the psychotropic drugs. Here I also acknowledge blame. Frantic to contain the misery of an unmoored Mother, we accepted without questions that psych drugs would help her. We did not go on the Internet and check on these drugs; we were barely treading water, and sleep deprived to boot.

Today the National Institute of Health (NIH) website carries bold warnings about the meds Abilify, Seroquel and Haldol.

- "Studies have shown that older adults with dementia who take anti-psychotics have an increased chance of death during treatment."
- "Older adults with dementia have an increased chance of stroke, mini-stroke or other severe side effects during treatment."
- "Not FDA approved for the elderly with dementia"

The warnings continue about unexplained elder deaths and how these meds are not to be prescribed for the elderly with stroke risk. Even now I'm flabbergasted that these drugs were given to Mother, regularly and in combination, without anyone on the medical staff mentioning the risk factors. That's not to say that we wouldn't have tried anything to alleviate Mother's terrors, in the way morphine is chosen to treat pain despite the risks. But at least we could've discussed the decision. And here's the thing, I don't think they really worked for Mother.

MY HOLISTIC APPROACH

Being in the hospital, however necessary and life saving, was a trial for all of us. Mother expressed this, in her incomplete verbal style, to Alex one listless afternoon beside her hospital bed. She attempted to tell him about her appointments with Dr. A in Seattle, of her comfort during their office visit. Halting in her explanations, she would look at me to complete her sentences. "We need more medicine like that here," she told her bedside audience.

As daughters, we each responded to Mother's physical and emotional needs from our personal resources. I took from my bevy of essential oils to help allay Mother's agitation.

Essential oils are to me the essence, the soul and the wisdom of a plant. They are distilled concentrates, which can waft a person away to the ether for a healing moment.* In his book "*Jitterbug Perfume*" Tom Robbins offers: "Smell is the sister of light, it is the left hand of the ultimate. It fastens the eternal to the temporal, This Side to That Side, and thus is highly sensitive." He characterizes

* This information comes from my love affair with essential oils and decades of experience. There are many excellent books available, as well as classes and other venues to learn about essential oils. The best way to explore the benefits of essential oils could be as simple as buying one and making the discovery personally.

scent as the last sense we let go of before death. Before "we sink into dream soup."

Invoking symmetry, we speculate that smell, that keeper of memory, could be our last surviving sense, because it is believed to have been one of our earliest. The olfactory system is an ancient and primitive structure. It is the only sensory system that does not have to pass through the thalamus; instead olfactory axons follow a pathway directly to the limbic system of our brain without being registered by the cerebral cortex. Other senses like sight and touch go through our conscious brain, to be recognized and sorted by our intelligence. Smell is literally on the fast track; it is the express train, with no stops at the thalamus. The aroma is absorbed through our nasal cavity into the olfactory receptors of our olfactory bulb. The small, easily absorbable molecules of essential oils then go to the limbic system, or the emotional center of our brain. Only a few chemically dangerous smells, like ammonia, are not sent to this subconscious part of our mind. How lovely: essential oils make a mad dash for the part of our brain where mood, creativity and motivation arise. The olfactory and limbic systems were created as unfettered partners. The limbic system, after olfactory stimuli, releases neurotransmitters like serotonin and endorphins, those happy brain juices.

Like herbs, all essential oils are not created equal. With the purest essential oils everything is done by hand, from the harvesting of the botanicals to the filling and labeling of the bottles. Extraction is best without chemicals like hexane or other synthetics. Little stands in the way of falsifying many essential oils, for other substances than the pure essential oil sometimes may not be detectable, even with the aid of a gas chromatograph. The truth remains that the way to insure quality oils is to know the source. I prefer certified organic or wild-crafted essential oils. Pure oils also come from boutique farmers, who use no chemicals but live outside the sphere of organic certification while making esoteric essential oils and saving rare species of botanicals.

Someone is feeling stressed and breathes in lavender. Like a good dice roll in the children's game "chutes and ladders," the lavender molecules slide quickly into the area where joy and fear are regulated. The neurotransmitter encephaline is released to produce a sense of well-being. Temper, rage and flight-or-fight also originate from this complicated limbic world: I like to soothe those unconscious sensations with bergamot or chamomile. Thus, those were the essential oils I whisked into my suitcase in Seattle and took to Memphis with me. I brought blue chamomile, lavender and citrus essential oils, which are suggested to be gentle enough for children. Oils consoling to children seemed to suit an elder brain fried by a stroke; the oils appeased the emotions and temper tantrums that accompanied such a disaster. I poured those oils and distilled water into an empty spray bottle, and I constantly spritzed the hospital rooms we inhabited to treat the hospital smells of fear, chemicals and adult diapers. The nurses would come into my mother's hospital room, raving about how good it smelled. I explained to several of them, Kizzie in particular, how to make such a mist, offering mini-essential oil classes in that bleached medical world. Mists are only one medium for essential oils. You can add essential oils to lotions or carrier oils (such as argan or avocado oil) to apply directly to your body; you can scent your home or office using a fragrance bowl of water and your favored essential oils, or you can find a wide choice of diffusers.

Ravinstara Aromatica essential oil, a strong antimicrobial, was my medicine. My mother and sister got "fever blisters" which we nursed with ravinstara.* We rubbed it on the glands of our neck areas to support lymphatic and immune health, to protect us from the bacteria coursing through the hospital. The clean aroma of ravintsara recalls eucalyptus, and as well as being a strong immune stimulant, it is a most powerful anti-viral essential oil. Consider ravintsara for canker sores, cold sores, herpes outbreaks, lymph nodes and shingles.

Clary sage is best known for getting us through rough psychological times, for its depression-relieving properties. Traditionally clary sage is used to assuage nervousness and paranoia, which were rampant in my mother's damaged neurons. It's also good for mature skin types. I would rub the oil on my mother's forehead when she got distressed and add it to lotions to massage her body for aches and bruises. Jumping the bed rails and landing with her body buckled on the floor had left Mother with some big blue repercussions. I patted her face with clary sage when she got emotionally out of control. She had skin wounds from all the tests, which I tended with helichrysum essential oil.

Helichrysum, with the botanical name Immortelle, holds sway as my favorite essential oil. Helichrysum is extracted by steam distillation from Italian straw flowers, those clutters of bright yellow blossoms that keep their shape and color when dried. Hence, they are also called Life Everlasting. This potent oil can be an effective

* As with all medicinal oils, first do a skin test to determine sensitivity. While some people may be able to use ravintsara directly on cold sores, others may need to mix it with shea butter or a few drops of carrier oil. A 50/50 mixture of ravintsara and carrier oil is a soothing topical combination for the misery of shingles. Use a warm compress with ravintsara on the neck for sore throats or swollen lymph nodes.

treatment for bruises, inflammations, couperose, mature skin and scars. Jeanne Rose, the famous herbalist, touts helichrysum as the best essential oil for scars with of its deep skin penetration. Since it may bolster cell regeneration and tissue rebuilding, I dabbed it on Mother's scabs from the EEG. The warm, woody aroma can be comforting for emotional bruising and stress. It is said to lessen effects of shock and fear, feelings rampant for Mother and her daughters. Life Everlasting spreads easily, and the essential oil reflects that gentle persistence, easing restlessness and offering patience, acceptance and forgiveness.

Essential oils existed as the physical, aromatic presentations of my personal prayers. If Tom Robbins is right, just before I die I may smell my mother's homemade rolls and remember love, or I may inhale the scent of sandalwood and feel harmony as I change worlds. I wanted Mother to have those same reassurances in the agony of that hospital world.

Chapter 14

HER FINAL DAYS

"The ideal death, I think, is what was the ideal Victorian death: You know, your grandchildren around you, a bit of sobbing — because, after all, tears are appropriate on a death bed — and you say goodbye to your loved ones."
Terry Patchett, author and AD patient

Memphis, February 2009

After playing pass-the-car-keys for weeks, Bev and I drove together to the Kenwood facility. We speculated on how Mother survived the night without the Adavin or Haldol. In the car with us we packed an extra chair, a better pillow, another lamp, and other decorations to make that bare bones room more livable. It was Thursday, Mother had spent one night at Kenwood, and Bev would fly back to California early Friday. However, the sisterly confluence would continue when Judy arrived late Friday night, for the weekend.

Shirley, Mother's night caregiver, greeted us with news of a good night. Bev and I thanked Shirley, opened the curtains to the weak winter light from the flowerless courtyard and soon met the rehab folks. Mother had slept through our attempts to feed her breakfast, but the therapists, humanely doing their job, tried to rouse Mother and sit her up in bed. Basically, Mother's somnolence shocked them. "What is she doing here?" they asked. "Why did the hospital discharge her?" I blamed the hospital meds, but Mother's lassitude disturbed them. They did their best and wished for a better response tomorrow. Mother melted back into her narcolepsy.

In the bleakness of the facility Bev and I sat on the bed on either side of Mother, talking across her freight-train snores. I asked Bev, petting Mother's boney arm, "What do you remember about her as a mother?"

Bev: "When I was a high school cheerleader, we had dinner before each game at one of the cheerleader's houses. Besides cooking, Mother made all the cheerleaders red half-slips. Remember when she was in her nylon and lace phase? She took the half-slips and turned them into some kind of centerpiece for the dinner table. Each of us got to take our slip from the centerpiece afterwards."

Me: "When I was pledging the high school sorority, the egg session was brutal. I came home crying, vowing to quit after gagging on raw eggs and having dozens cracked on my head. Mother knew how much I wanted to belong with the popular girls and encouraged me to stick it out. She showed me the nightshirt she had just made for my sorority big sister. She had stitched Sigma Sigma in big letters on this pin-striped nightshirt."

Like the basketball Mother played in high school and college, where only three dribbles were allowed and the basketball had to be passed to another team member, Bev and I tossed our memories over Mother. Mother stayed asleep, not even playing defense, but we challenged her to get back in the game.

"She took a just-baked warm cake every Friday when she went to do the weekly payroll at The Place."

"Camping toast in the skillet."

"Standing on the cedar chest at the end of her bed while she pinned up the hem of a new skirt she was making."

"Pork chops and gravy for breakfast." One, two, three bounces, pass the ball.

"Her flowerbeds! She dug up ferns everywhere they traveled."

"And every pastel color of those tiny little roses. She put them on Daddy's pillow when he had cancer."

In spite of our verbal enticements, Mother spent most of the day in what seemed to be a semi-comatose state. We fed her liquids by spoon and tiny bites of pureed food because she was having trouble swallowing. But we'd seen this before, seen her come back: after all she had been heavily medicated for over three weeks. Still, the Kenwood staff was alarmed.

When it came time for Shirley's arrival, Bev told our slumbering Mother, "I'm going home to California tomorrow to see Mitchell and Taylor, but I'll come back later. Maybe by then you'll be feeling better. They'll have you talking and walking around in no time."

I stood apart, leaning against the beige wall, my hands in my pockets. I said softly to Bev, "You have to tell her good-bye. Just in case."

Like a sudden storm rolling into a Memphis summer day Bev began talking to Mother, crying, telling her what a wonderful Mother she was, hugging her. I slipped out of the room.

The next morning Alex took Bev to the airport at 5 a.m., getting more stars for his crown in heaven, as Mother liked to say. I headed to Kenwood to relieve Shirley. On the way I checked my voicemail. A message from the Physician's Assistant (PA) at Kenwood relayed that Mother's chest x-ray showed pneumonia.

The PA suggested antibiotics. Mother didn't stir when I kissed her forehead, opened the curtains, and hugged Shirley good-bye for the day. It was 7:30 in the morning and my mind was racing. For the record, I had appreciated my previous interactions with the PA; thus, I expected a friendly communication with her when she entered the stark room.

Quickly I said, "no antibiotics." It was already specified on the medical power of attorney I had given Kenwood.

The Physician's Assistant, stout and overworked, ignored me, barreling ahead. "The pneumonia is only a very small spot on your mother's lung. The antibiotics are strong and will probably clear it up quickly. Then we'll do another x-ray, and if her lung looks good, we'll take her to a hospital near Kenwood for tests. You and your sisters really should prepare for a long haul. She can get over this pneumonia."

"Take her to a hospital for tests? She's barely awake. We don't want to stress her with another ambulance ride. No, I'm not putting her on antibiotics." My voice was shaking, maybe my whole body, as I stood stiffly at the foot of Mother's hospital bed.

The PA was unyielding, her face stern: "You need to listen better," she reprimanded. "I didn't say we'd take her to the hospital right away." Then she lectured me on how many caregivers died first, how I needed to relax, pace myself, put Mother on antibiotics.

"No," I said, suddenly aware that I was not going to let Mother die in this smelly enclosure. "And I'm taking my mother home today." Mother had been through enough, and I had the power to make her transition more comfortable. I would take her home to die in her sleep like she had always prayed.

The PA was aghast. "That won't be possible," she fumbled. "It's Friday and you won't be able to get the equipment delivered to your house until Monday. Give your mother the weekend to see if she gets better. You won't be able to get her out of here before next week. How will you take care of her at home? She needs a lot of care." She had more to say before she left the room. Mother remained in her stupor.

I thought to myself, "You just watch me, I AM taking Mother home today."

Looking for a miracle, slightly teary, I called Linda, my red-headed best friend from high school now a Hospice chaplain, soliciting advice about what to do to get Mother home. As teen-agers we spent the night at each other's houses, went to each other's churches, studied (or not) together, and even ran against each other for Student Council office. I was in her wedding when she married the honor society and football star. Our sons were born only a month apart, though in different time zones. She went to seminary and became a Southern Baptist minister, which did not go over well in Memphis. Women were not welcomed into Baptist pulpits. She became a chaplain at St. Jude's Children's Hospital, and was now a hospice chaplain. Linda's compassion consoled me, and she gave me a list: we needed a signed release by Mother's doctor or the facility doctor, to sign Mother up for Hospice, a "prescription" for a hospital bed and anything else necessary, like oxygen and meds, and an ambulance to take her home. I called Bev, where she was having barbeque (for breakfast?) in the Memphis airport. I rattled through the details. In spite of the DNR, Bev hesitated about not giving Mother the antibiotics, but she agreed about taking Mother home. I called Judy, at her desk at work. She said okay and that she would get to Memphis about eleven that night, making the long drive from Chattanooga after she got off work. And so it began, calls to get a doctor's signature, papers from hospice to Kenwood, papers faxed back to hospice, papers for me as power of attorney to sign, hospital equipment ordered, an antibiotic prescription, Chaplain Linda pushing through the paperwork and getting her friends at hospice to make an extra effort to get Mother home.

Somewhere during that hectic morning, as I stood at the nurses' station, reading medical legalese, the PA said to me "I hope it wasn't something I said."

"This is not about you," I replied fiercely, sliding another stack of papers toward her. "This is about my Mother. I'm doing what she would want. I'm taking her home."

I called in favors from Mother's village of admirers to move furniture out of Mother's study and into the garage. Meanwhile, Mother slept through the fury of activity required to get her out of Kenwood. Checking on delivery time for the hospital bed, I found that paperwork had gotten lost in the melee. Calling Aunt Lottye and Uncle Jim to come and stay with Mother, I handled the problem.

In phenomenal time, between the morning when Bev left and the evening when Judy arrived, despite the protests of the nursing home PA, then a slight glitch in the equipment delivery, and thanks to the determination of Chaplain Linda, Mother was on her way home. As I met the home equipment man at Magnolia Village around seven o'clock, Lottye Kaye saw Mother off on that final ambulance ride, tucking an extra blanket around Mother's frangible body. When the big hospital equipment truck pulled into the tight dead-end lane behind Mother's condo, there was already an even bigger truck right across from us for a neighbor who was having a mattress delivered. I put sheets on the hospital bed, signed more papers, and was shown how to use the oxygen equipment. Then into that fray of big trucks, with the oxygen still being set up inside, came the ambulance bearing Mother.

Mother was zonked as the EMTs tried unsuccessfully to maneuver the inflexible gurney down the compact hallway, lifted her off the gurney and carried her skin-and-bones frame into her own space once again. She opened her eyes widely and looked around. I had hung Aunt E's paintings on the wall facing Mother's bed, put up a picture of Daddy, and a poem Soren had written about her that she had framed years ago. For weeks in the hospital she cried, fought, pleaded, demanded, kicked, screamed, and even offered me $5 to get her home. How could we be astounded that, like most of her life, dying, too, was on her terms?

Shirley, coming for the night shift, found the Magnolia Condo Village after a couple of calls, navigating through the tree-lined streets. We assessed Mother's needs, and I went to the drug store to get a rubber suction bulb and liquid dropper, plus more diapers. I found everything I needed in the baby section. Irony or the complete circle, I wasn't sure. By the time Judy arrived in the last hours of that significant day, Shirley was settled into Mother's big chair, watching over her. It had been a long day, life fast forwarded into streaks of vibrant, moving light, colors rapidly rearranging the scene. Looking back on that Friday, it was accompanied by strange music in my head, airplanes heading west, sisters hugging, everyone's steps in double and triple time, me making a dozen trips back and forth to the car carrying lamps and bedding, Mother rolling down halls on a gurney, big trucks rolling in and out of Magnolia Village, until Mother was restored to her final heart's desire.

The next morning, Saturday, Judy and I sat at Mother's dining room table, previous meals replaced by scary stacks of papers, when the hospice nurse knocked on the front door. She arrived to dispense sympathy, information, and comfort meds. Judy and I were allowed the time we needed to ask any questions. Dutiful daughters, we took notes about each med and started a log. Hospice would provide us with a visiting nurse, a social worker, an emergency phone number to call, and, of course, Chaplain Linda. The nurse made sure we understood to call hospice and not 911 if Mother had an emergency. While open and direct, she had no exact answers about how long Mother might live. Mother's vitals, her breathing, her heart, her skin and nail tone looked good, the nurse told us. She again reminded us, there's no reason for your mother to suffer. All the while, Mother continued her slumber.

Judy hung a pretty banner across the windows beside Mother's hospital bed, pinning all the cards Mother had received on a big yellow satin ribbon. I went to Whole Foods and bought organic baby food, vegetable juice, fish oil, and organic broths. Chaplin Linda brought over bags of food for us, especially vegetarian choices for me. What a relief to be away from institutionalized medicine and awful hospital food. We were exploring the daily needs of a dying Mother, the small and large rites of caretaking at home. Mother, in some ways, looked remarkable. Her skin was rosy; the ugly burn that had covered her thumb when she first got to the hospital and the scabs left on her forehead by the EEG had healed. On Sunday morning Judy found all the burial papers, and we sorted through more bank and annuity statements, as well as over-due bills. Then we made our affectionate good-byes.

Later on that Sunday after Judy left, the doorbell rang. There stood Aunt Lottye Kaye and Uncle Jim, bringing back the chair that I had left at Kenwood.

"It was coming apart, and I fixed it," Uncle Jim showed me proudly.

I warned them that I didn't know if Mother would wake up, as we went into her new habitude. Much to the delight of all of us in

Mother's room, Mother awoke and joined in a conversation with Aunt Lottye Kaye. When Lottye smiled and asked Mother something, Mother was able to make a few words, struggling with the effort, then trail off with "j-ja-j-je-j." Then she would laugh gleefully! Laugh with a joy long absent from her life. The conversation went like that, questions or statements from Lottye Kaye, Mother managing a few words, trailing off with j-ja-ja-j and getting the biggest kick out of it.

I walked Lottye Kaye and Uncle Jim to the front door, thanked and hugged them, and by the time I got back to Mother's room, she was already asleep. I straightened her covers, kissed her cheek, and called Judy with "You won't believe what just happened!" Surely, we had turned some corner.

Bev emailed friends, neighbors and relatives for us: *Currently, Marilyn is at home with Mother. We encourage you to come by and see Mother. Possibly this will be a chance for you to remember fond times with Mother and say your goodbyes.*

My time in Memphis with Mother was dear to me. There were moments when she made me laugh and other times when I couldn't stop crying. I feel so blessed to have had Mom out here at our home for the Christmas holidays. It was such a joyous experience, and I'm so thankful for that uninterrupted time with her.

I recalled again "Summons to Memphis," Peter Taylor's book about adult children being called to Memphis because of a parental crisis. Like the book, I was seeped in Memphis because of my parent, percolating in aunts, cousins, and friends from high school, followed around by old family photos. I took care of Mother's daily needs, keeping her mouth and lips moist, giving her comfort meds, consoling her, and singing to her, my lips humming right next to her ear. The ole church songs popped into my head: "it's me, it's me, it's me, oh Lord, standin' in the need of prayer." Appropriately I changed it to "its Lou, it's Lou, it's Lou, oh Lord." I massaged essential oils onto her temples.

Sitting beside Mother as she weakened, it no longer mattered if she knew who I was. The agony had ended of her looking at me in the hospital, baffled, trying to figure me out by asking "are your parents alive?" or "do you have any children?" Back in her own home Mother and I serenely passed the hours, undisturbed. Every day was about the minute acts of care giving, the sacrament of details. I did everything I could for the moment: changed her diapers, gave her a suppository for fever, put moisturizer on her dry lips, anointed her with essential oils and rose day cream, turned her on her side, put the oxygen mask on her, and sang her a hymn or two. "When my way grows drear, Precious Lord, linger near, when my life is almost gone." Then I put on my ear buds. Dr. John sang: "life is short, yall."

I emailed friends: *All I want to say, and you all know this, I want the Nevilles rocking out with Dancing Jones during my last days. Even if I seem to sleep through it. Sure it doesn't fit my mother's religious life, and I do, indeed, quote scripture to her; I can call up the 23rd Psalm and my sister Judy has taped Bible verses on the wall beside Mother's bed. But please, for me, crank up the music, and dance me into the next world.*

The hospice social worker had a cadre of questions to get to know us. She looked at her notes, "Your father owned the Esso station on Highland? Really? I always got my car fixed there when I went to Memphis State." Daddy's business was about half a mile from the university. "Do you remember Eddie?"

"Of course I remember Eddie." We were sitting in the living room talking, while Mother lay dormant in her world of private dreams. “Eddie was homeless and slept in a car on Daddy’s property. Daddy would give him work, or money, or food. Eddie was a fixture on Highland.” We didn’t need to say that Eddie was black.

“When I was in college, I hung out at the pubs on Highland. I saw Eddie around. I collected money and talked to people and got him a place to stay.” Her social worker roots had sprouted early. “But it didn’t work out. He went back to living in the car.”

And my parents went back to looking after him.

Linda also made official chaplain visits in addition to her thoughtful outpourings of friendship, her red hair a halo of warmth. Her susurrus and faith surely reached Mother.

As we stood beside Mother, holding her limp hand, I said to Linda, “dying isn’t easy.”

The phone would ring, neighbors would appear at the front door, church ladies came on canes. “Get well, Lou, and come live at Mason Gardens next door to me. We’ll have such a good time.” I would leave them alone with Mother. On the way out, they paused, flush with dolor and respect, “She was a fine Christian woman.” “She was a good neighbor.” “She was a great Sunday School teacher.”

I continued to pet Mother, to drop a swallow of vegetable juice on her tongue, to tell her how much I loved her. I rubbed her arms and hands with lotion, crushed her pills in applesauce, wrote down when she was restless and needed meds, and at night would help Shirley change and bathe Mother. With Shirley I expressed gratitude for the succor Mother was receiving, for how everything was unfolding. Shirley said it could be the prayers that Mother had prayed her whole life; I could sense Mother’s prayers for other people, endless hours spent in thanks and supplication, coming back to bless and protect her now, the encircling power of her belief.

The days passed. Mother's vitals were strong, her lungs sounded clear, her skin was full of color. But her brain had slipped away, as well as her physical abilities. She had gone from constant chatter about her other world (are the kids in bed, are the doors locked, where's Howard, you're so mean, my sister is waiting for me, do you have a car to get me out of here?) to having no more words. She seemed at last in eternal quiet.

One afternoon while I sat by Mother's bed watching movies on my computer, Mother awoke, up to her ole trickery of getting out of bed. But something, some encounter with life, pain, or death, horrified her. Her eyes were truly fearful as she clung to me, and I enfolded and kissed her. With mellifluous words I promised her that she was home and it was going to be all right. She only got quiet after I gave her some morphine and haldol. After that Mother never came back, her eyes open and staring blankly into space, her breath slowing, her mouth agape. I used the baby dropper to give her literal drops of water and juice, her swallowing now gone, and with a tiny pink sponge swab and a spritz of herbal tincture I cleansed her mouth.

Shirley knocked on my bedroom door in the middle of the night. "You better come." Grace came to our Mother and she stopped breathing. No struggle and just as she had always told us, she died in her sleep at home.

I called the hospice number requesting a nurse. Shirley and I embraced tearfully one last time. I sat beside Mother's body until the nurse arrived in the pitch dark. The funeral home men came in suits and politeness to get Mother, and she was taken out on a gurney, much like she had come back home earlier. By then our family was making airline reservations from Maryland, California and Ohio.

Everything else I needed to do had to wait for daylight, so I made myself some breakfast and emailed friends and relatives: *Early this morning my mom peacefully left this world for a better one. During her traumatic stay in the hospital when she was so confused and bothered, she would call my dad, "Howard! HOWARD WALLS!" Finally, as she wanted him, Elois and Jack, her parents, and other friends who had left her, I began to say, "He's in heaven." "She's in heaven." Then my mother paused thoughtfully and told me firmly, in her somewhat garbled communication, that she was going to get a cab to take her to heaven. It was an easy cab ride for her this morning. Her life was a blessing to many and I was lucky to be her daughter.*

One of the practical gifts Mother left us was planning her own funeral. She had paid for it ahead of time when Daddy died, selecting her casket and other arrangements. Friends have found their credit cards maxed out to pay for a parent's funeral, have wondered how and where to honor the loved one. Not only was it easier on us, the weary daughters, but Mother got to have the funeral she wanted.

Mother had chosen to be buried in the peach suit with the tiny iridescent pearls on the collar, which she had worn to her first granddaughter's wedding. She loved that suit, and how she must have blended with the peach highlights of her sofa and loveseat when she passed through her living room wearing it. She would never have thought of the hue as fleshy, she simply preferred subtle when it came to decorating. Just as she had picked out clothes for Daddy every day when he was alive and left them spread on the bed for him, I put out her suit. It dissolved into the subdued tints of the flowered bedspread. The matching blouse was not to be found.

Never fear, there were alternatives in her closet: ivory, blush, and other innocent shades offered their Sunday finery for her final gathering. Her bed, where she and Daddy had slept together for years, where we had sat for conversations and where she fretted through seemingly endless, sleepless nights, was quickly covered with blouses and accessories. Obviously, she did not realize the dangerous gaps she left in the hands of her most flamboyant daughter. Soon, however, I had a tasteful outfit she would approve. She wouldn't need any shoes, but I grabbed a pair of red, fuzzy socks. She was always cold natured and shivering, probably worsened by her thyroid problems. On family car trips in the 1950s, where the air conditioner hung below the dash board with no vents to regulate the air flow and blew directly on her shotgun, map-reading seat, she covered herself with a scratchy blanket in the white heat of summer. At my house she camped in the garnet chair beside the amber glow of the gas fireplace. She was chilled her whole life, initiating the thermostat wars when any of us visited her. She would push the temperature up, and once she was in bed, nieces and daughters, sweating in the dead of winter, would sneak in to lower the thermostat.

In the hushed halls of the funeral home, I handed the ensemble for Mother's closing act to the decorous man with the consoling smile. Tentatively, I gave him the bright ruby socks. Yes, I knew she was dead, without sensations, but I explained to the somber-suited gentleman who delicately accepted her clothes, "Her feet were always cold."

All kindness, his tones soothing like Mother's color palette, "We'll put them on her." Nothing could faze him there in the refined atmosphere of death.

In spite of a bizarre spring snow, relatives, our friends from high school and college, Mother's neighbors, and church folks came to the visitation at the funeral home. Mother's "husk" was lovely, surrounded by her favorite shades of pink and peach, and by elaborate flower arrangements, many matching her chosen decor. Judy's daughters made the photo boards, showing Mother as fresh-faced youth, a wide-eyed bride, and a doting grandmother. Everyone said how sweet Mother was and many cried at the finality, about how much they would miss her. They came with walkers, with tales, from long drives across other southern state lines, after sharing a lifetime that brought us standing around her casket, our own hair now silver, our hearts strangely both empty and full.

Mother had given Norma Sue, a pretty older cousin whom I worshipped a little when she was a teen-ager, her first baby-sitting job. I was just an infant. "I was so nervous" Norma explained, "that I cleaned the whole house. I wanted to do everything right. You were a good baby," she added as an afterthought.

"Really?" I was wearing a long skirt and simple jacket, which would have made Mother proud. "Mother said they had to put me on goat's milk because I was so allergic."

Norma Sue snickered, "Oh! You spit up!" Trouble at any early age. Doomed to disrupt.

At Mother's home the morning of the funeral I said to Soren as he ate his breakfast alone at the dining room table, "Bev's getting cranky."

Wisely he pronounced, looking up from his laptop, "she's sad." That said it all.

The snow came down, after following Mother across the country to visit her daughters for her last holidays, and continued through the Memphis night. For the first time in ten years all of Mother's generations congregated at the same time. It was barbeque for every meal, the food and drink delivered by family and friends in large pans and ice chests with wheels. Southern traditions are potent in times of loss, thick with friendship, red meat, and desserts. Though the courteous and efficient funeral director had called to see if we wanted to cancel the service or burial because of the snow and ice, the chapel was full of Mother's adoring companions. Linda's daughter sang beautifully. The granddaughters were overcome with tears, but all of the grandkids stood strong for the difficult task of reading from the Laura-designed, grandkids-written birthday book "85 Reasons Why We Love Grandma Lou." Soren was last, being the oldest, reading his Corinthians-inspired tribute, but all six of them painted a word picture of Mother's generosities and intimate grandmother moments.

The men of Mother's family were the pallbearers, grandsons, sons-in-law, and grandsons-in-law, wearing coats of wool and leather, with small roses on their lapels; they lifted the white casket reverently. Each man placed the rose on the casket as they walked away.

At the graveside, a white tent protecting family from the snow, Brent, the articulate minister from Mother's church quoted Mark Twain. "When someone dies it takes years to realize what all we've lost." We had those mournful discoveries yet to face.

Even without Mother's direction, we pulled off a reception with more barbeque and banana pudding. Later back in Mother's home, just the sisters and our families, we let loose, laughing and talking story. We held our own private wake, four generations spilling out from the kitchen and crowded around the table, as with all of Mother's best gatherings.

Chapter 15

SCIENCE FOR CAREGIVERS

"There are only four kinds of people in this world. Those who have been caregivers. Those who are currently caregivers. Those who will be caregivers. And those who will need caregivers."
Rosalyn Carter, Board of Directors for The Rosalynn Carter Institute for Caregiving, and former First Lady

Standing at the foot of my mother's bed in the Kenwood facility, the physician's assistant lectured me. "Your mother could live a long time. You have to pay attention and listen to me. You're not listening! Do you know how many caregivers die before the patient? Thirty percent!"

About one thing, she was right: I wasn't listening. I was planning Mother's escape from that small room. I didn't care how many caregivers died first. That was not my worry, an attitude probably commonplace among caregivers. Most caregivers are not thinking about the possibly of being a caregiver for a long time. The focus is on the crisis *du jour*, the latest test results, or the loss of yet another parental function.

As Mother faded away, I ignored those statistics of doom. However, the results of a 2003 study at Ohio State University about caregivers re-enforced the PA's warning. The researchers discovered a significant deterioration in the health of caregivers when compared to a similar group of non-caregivers. And here's the truly disturbing finding: caregivers had a 63 percent higher death rate than the control group. Before the end of the six-year study, 70 percent of the caregivers died and had to be replaced.[1] According to a 2015 National Alliance of Caregivers and AARP report, nearly 15,000,000 unpaid (most likely translation: family) Americans care for someone with AD or dementia.[2] In 2004, a study performed by the University of California's Department of Psychiatry reported that family caregiving can take as much as ten years from a caregiver's life.[3]

In spite of these dire studies, caring for a sick or dying family member can also be a gift. For many it brings redemption from earlier family conflicts, as well as the fulfillment of knowing that family is being treated with care and respect. Many caregivers have said it was precious to spend such a life-altering time with someone dear.

STRESS

Taking care of family contains many rewards, especially the opportunity to give back to a loving parent. The result of the daily overload of stress, however, can bring physical and psychological challenges. When I was taking care of Mother, I would remember the cliché, "That which doesn't kill you, makes you stronger." Honestly, when it comes to stress, that consolation isn't true. Short–term, stress might not kill you, but rather than making one stronger, it disrupts sleep, increases nervousness, depletes the immune system, and untreated, can cause chronic and acute illnesses. Some of those illnesses can, actually, kill you. Risk of stroke is especially pernicious and was most pronounced among men, especially African-American men.[4]

Daily coping balances precariously against the disappearing pieces of the beloved. Caregivers contend with out-of-control tasks, personal imperfections whether physical or emotional, and perhaps financial strain. This burden for family caregivers is not without consequences. Reactions can exhibit as isolation from friends and social gatherings; as issues like depression or substance abuse; or become physical problems such as constant pain or high blood pressure.

Much has been written to help caregivers. Some are simple reminders like exercise, eating well, and taking a break; more complicated problems such as financial and legal planning may require professional assistance. Of course, some of those ideas for coping can sound like a fantasy. "Now, Mom, don't wander off or start a kitchen fire while I'm out exercising. I know you understand that I need some relief from watching you act like a rebellious child. Wait, don't throw that vase at me!" Still, it is essential to recognize limits. Caregivers definitely need to vent, problem-solve or grieve with someone trusted. Perhaps family and friends are willing to listen, but don't be surprised if you require a professional.

Look for local help as well as finding assistance from national organizations. Alzheimer's Association groups have organized outings for patients and their caregivers. In some places, local museums provide a safe gathering for those with dementia and their caregivers. Art, with no requirements for short-term memory or rational explanations, can offer patients and their companions an outlet. Another idea involves reserving tables at a coffee shop during slow hours. Both caregivers and their charges can comfortably meet with those who understand the situation. A change of scenery and communication may go a long way in righting a day gone wrong. While such opportunities may alleviate stress for a little while, the truth of caregiving remains a commitment tinged with the probability of major health consequences.

BOTANICALS

Stress takes an enormous toll on the adrenals, where the flight or fight mechanism arises to provide energy for functioning during times of pressure. As the adrenals become depleted, cortisol increases, sleep is compromised and the immune system weakened. It doesn't require a professional to anticipate the outcome of that combination. Chronic stress cascades into anxiety. If uncurbed, stress can lead to burn-out and illness.

Botanicals thrive all over the world, and some may even offer adrenal support. Before airplanes or clinical research, ancient peoples recognized herbs that gave them strength through the crushing era of killer tigers (the ultimate in fight or flight) or freezing winters. In each part of the world plants had to develop a means of survival in bleak terrain and harsh conditions, and those plant protections were passed on to humans as flavonoids. This array of botanicals provided what traditional cultures needed: stamina and physical coping mechanisms against the elements, plus support for immunity and fertility. Such plants were an integral part of ethnic medicine for many centuries. Each culture had such a native plant: rhodiola in Siberia, ginseng in China, ashwaganda in India, maca in South America. Today these plants are called adaptogens. Adaptogen is a non-medical definition for a non-toxic normalizer believed to support the adrenal glands and endocrine system. Traditional herbalists categorize them as herbal tonics. These plants can increase the body's resistance to adverse conditions, giving the mechanism and energy to keep humans functioning during stress.

In this age of the availability of plants from all over the planet, a plethora of adaptogens can be found on shelves in local co-ops or natural health stores. My personal favorite is rhodiola, botanical name *rhodiola rosea* in honor of its red root. Originally found in Russia, Siberia, Asia, Alaska and other frigid climates, mythology claims rhodiola gave Vikings their strength. Signifiying fertility, brides carried rhodiola as a wedding bouquet.[5] Rhodiola was a well-kept Russian secret, used to increase the endurance of their athletes: it can shorten recovery time after physical exertion and has low toxicity.[6] Human studies show that rhodiola increases alertness and decreases fatigue; it is a free radical scavenger, thus enhancing antioxidant defenses and protecting against illness.[7] Rhodiola can also relieve irritability and insomnia. For physicians working the night shift, it reduced mental fatigue.[8] When taken by young military cadets who went for 24 hours without sleep, the participants' cognitive test scores showed improvement in both mental processing and short term memory.[9] Perhaps rhodiola can reduce burn-out and enhance mood, including support against anxiety.[10] All of these benefits could translate into positive affects for the challenges faced by caregivers.

Maca (*Lepidium meyenii*) is grown high in the mountains of Peru and other South American countries, where the plant has to adjust to high altitudes. As an adaptogen, maca proffers similar advantages: support for withstanding the brain-fogginess, exhaustion and sleepiness of care giving.[11] A Chinese herb, astragalus, has been used against the common cold and upper respiratory infections because of its anti-viral properties.[12] Studies show astragalus can activate the white blood cells and macrophages of the immune system.[13]

The Chinese will pay high prices for American ginseng (*Panax quinquefolis*); thus, this slow-growing plant has been thoughtlessly, even criminally harvested. In addition to its neuroprotective qualities, American ginseng may decrease blood pressure, as well as blood glucose and insulin levels.[14] Remembering the increased stroke risk for caregivers, ethically harvested American ginseng may be worth the extra expense.

Reishi medicinal mushroom (*Ganoderma lucidum*) guards the immune system.[15] This is my personal happy pill. Pictures of this sacred mushroom have been found from as far back as 3500 B.C. Monks grew reishi mushrooms on an isolated island to ensure the Emperor's longevity and immortality. These same monks took this woody mushroom to aid their practice of meditation. Current science has identified constituents such as polysaccharides and beta-glucans: these may increase the body's antioxidants, and up the T-cells, natural killer cells and macrophages in the immune system.[16] Reishi mushrooms may also protect against liver disease[17] and diabetes;[18] however, reishi is most studied for its anti-viral properties.[19] All those mechanisms support a healthy life, if not immortality. They also speak directly to a caregiver's physical challenges. Cordyceps is another medicinal mushroom, which provides respiratory and lung support.[20] Look for shitake mushrooms in the produce department of your grocery store and add them to your favorite dishes for immune enhancement and a nutty taste. Mushrooms are best cooked, rather than eaten raw, to release the most medicinal benefits.

Holy basil or tulsi (*Ocimum sanctum*), not to be confused with culinary basil, remains a sacred herb in India. Long revered in

Ayurvedic medicine, Holy Basil relaxes the central nervous system.[21] Unlike other adaptogens, Holy Basil favors bedtime. It could provide a much-needed assist for a good's night sleep and pleasant dreams, all the while buttressing those worn-out adrenals.

With adrenals rebooted, cortisol lessens and sleep may come more easily. However, herbs can affect each person differently, and you may to need try several adaptogens to find the one that suits you best. As always, consult your medical practitioner about these botanicals and all health issues. I am not a doctor, nor am I prescribing. Talking to a nutritionist, herbalist or naturopathic doctor can assist in navigating those rows of bottles, which taunt an overwhelmed customer. It's important to find brands that are trustworthy. Let me remind you again: "All herbs are <u>not</u> created equal." As with food, reading supplement labels is necessary.

<u>IMMUNITY</u>

Although caregivers may say, "I don't have time to get sick," that doesn't save them from illness. Time to call up some familiar nutrients to support the immune system. Choose colorful vegetables and fruits for antioxidant and anti-inflammatory upkeep. Feed the vitamin D receptors in the immune system. Deficiency in vitamin D is associated with increased autoimmunity as well as an increased susceptibility to infection.[22] In a study of vitamin D and inflammation, the highest levels of vitamin D were required for maximum immune response.[23] The hindrances to getting vitamin D in food, and even in sunlight, make it a candidate for supplementation, and an inexpensive choice, at that. Again, your health care provider would be the best source for how much vitamin D to take.

Microflora contributes to a strong immune system. In fact, with 70-80 percent of the immune system residing in the G.I. tract,[24] the health of the entire body is modulated by the complex array of flora there. Good bacteria fight inflammation and infection, especially inflammation in the G.I. tract.

ANXIETY

Maintaining mental health is a complicated labyrinth with hallways of environmental stress, corners of family disappointments, or an open space lit by success. From feelings of worry and edginess to full-blown panic, anxiety has staked a claim on modern lives. Everyone feels anxious at one time or another, although caregivers have a particular burden. Women especially fall prey: anxiety is two to three times more common in women, increased in perimenopause, and about two-thirds of caregivers are women.[25] Caregiving elongates the cycle: inner turmoil, irritability, trouble concentrating, sleep problems, perhaps health issues. Anxiety can be a short-term state or a long-term trait. No magic bullet exists at this time to fix either generalized or specific anxiety. Talk therapy, meditation, medications and exercise all have soothed anxious souls.

Nutrition currently is being examined as a piece of the puzzle. Both animal and human studies have verified that being well nourished helps decrease anxiety and fortifies the ability to deal with stressful situations.[26] A New Zealand study elaborated on this idea when scientists found that on days young adults ate more fruits and vegetables, they reported an enhanced sense of curiosity and creativity. This added to the growing evidence that a diet rich in fruits and vegetables is related to greater happiness, life satisfaction, and positive affect.[27] A daily diet high in fruits and vegetables certainly will provide the antioxidants, vitamins and minerals needed to improve your mood.

Although scientists call this the very beginning of understanding how the brain works, they now think that neural circuitry involving the nucleus accumbens, the amygdala and the hippocampus underlie anxiety.[28] All are neighbors in the brain and communicate in response to stress, a kind of emotional Bermuda Triangle. The hippocampus makes memories, especially about events and facts. A memory alone might trigger anxiety. The hippocampus sends its information to other regions of the brain, including the amygdala, the alarmist of the brain. It doesn't require a brain surgeon to see the connection between stress, anxiety and brain function. Stress creates a loop in the brain, a circle arising from poor sleep, poor nutrition or emotional distress. This leads to the brain's decreased ability to concentrate. The circle continues with worry, as focus and learning take a hit. Cortisol rises, and the hippocampus loses neurons and volume. Meanwhile the amygdala has the whole body on high alert, and the nucleus accumbens, the brains's addict, is looking for comfort in sugar, coffee or some other favored drug.

Studies promote the role of nutrition in hippocampal strength. All omega-3 fatty acids are concentrated in the brain, but DHA especially has been confirmed to offer new neurons to fight against the stress cycle.[29] One study of post-traumatic stress disorder, self-described as a "novel preventative strategy," found that omega-3s, particularly DHA, worked in the clearance of fear memories from the hippocampus.[30]

Those anthocyanins in a blueberry smoothie would be useful and delicious to protect the hippocampus and stimulate new cell creation. They defend against neuron excitotoxicity, a hyperresponsiveness that's a piece of the anxiety puzzle.[31] The anthocyanins in frozen blueberries maintain their potency for three to six months, making that smoothie a year-round protective treat!

People experiencing anxiety have been found to have lower levels of magnesium. Magnesium, a calming mineral deficient in most diets, has the ability to "suppress hippocampal kindling" according to a study, and may guard against stress hormones entering the brain.[32] The amygdala signals the entire body, creating tight muscles, increased sensitivities and insomnia. Magnesium can relax these symptoms. A calcium-magnesium supplement taken at night may also defend against muscle cramps that interrupt sleep.

THE MICROBIOME

Ancient cultures believed that the center of the self was located in the belly. The Chinese word for belly means "mind place," and the Japanese word for belly, "hara," represents the seat of understanding. Those concepts were early articulations of the gut-brain axis. One study put it this way: gut inflammation can increase anxiety.[33] Enter the microbiome.

Early microbiome studies examined mice. Researchers described two groups of mice; one was "garrulous and risk-taking," the other shy and anxious. The microflora of the two groups were switched and their behaviors reversed.[34] Bold mice became tenuous, quiet mice talkative.

Like the science of emotion, microbiome research is in its infancy. Expect new discoveries in both fields of study, but consider what currently is acknowledged. Anxiety disorders are common in patients with disturbed gut flora. In a 2011 human study, 30 days of the probiotics *Lactobacillus heleveticus* and *Bifidobacteria longum* netted less anxiety.[35] One mechanism for these effects may be that some microbes make significant contributions to the production of GABA and other anxiety-reducing neurotransmitters, as well as increasing tryptophan, DHA and serotonin.[36] Those same scientists remind us, "We simply cannot view the gut-brain-microbiota axis as isolated from diet or the context of its macro and micronutrients."[37] Again, no magic pill exists as a panacea. Healthy food choices are necessary for a healthy home for the microbiome. While the studies on probiotics are promising, much is left to learn, especially about the over-use of a single strain vs. the synergy of a profile of microbiota. My suggestion if you do decide to take a probiotic supplement: a diverse profile of bacteria may be your best choice until more knowledge about the workings of specific strains is understood.

A HOLISTIC APPROACH

The meshing of anxiety's symptoms, causes and solutions creates a complicated netting sometimes difficult to unravel. Herbs and essential oils offer symptom relief, while talk therapy may quiet an aroused amygdala. Healthy food choices of fruits, vegetables and fish can assist the hippocampus. Caring for this condition calls for a holistic approach including a variety of treatments and asking for help with your caregiving commitments.

Stress, especially for caregivers, cannot be eliminated, and some unease may be impetus for the completion of a task or for barreling through the latest AD dilemma. The existential philosophers believed that anxiety is to be accepted as a part of the human condition. Perhaps a well-nourished body and brain support the ability to handle the triggers that set off anxiety and illness.

Chapter 16

TEARS FOR MY MOTHER

"Your grief is the substitute for their presence on earth. Your grief is their presence on earth."

Andres Holleran, Grief

Memphis, Spring 2009

After the funeral, our numbers dwindled to three sisters. Ahead was the task of dismantling the possessions of Mother's life. Of making decisions about the possessions held dear by her, all the uncollectables she accumulated.

The limited window of time we had together exacerbated the process. In those few days we began to decide who got what. Even in the best of families, it can be messy. (Into a paper bag, like flour-coated chicken parts, shake fairness, ego, memories, unresolved family issues and money.) We made a plan. An expert assessed the valuable things. One hundred dollars well spent. (Deep fry in sorrow.) With each of our choices, the amount would be entered on the ledger. (Drain on tear-soaked tissues.)

We went through Mother's overstuffed closets, draping ourselves in scarves. We covered her bed with skirts and blouses and blazers and tried them on, walking around in our underwear, putting on this dress or that sweater. We all took pajamas, Mother was such a pajama gal, and collected for the granddaughters. Her shoes startled and bemused me: purple suede pumps and low-heeled black patent leather, stylin' shoes barely worn. The purple suedes knocked me out, but her size eleven narrow outsized my fat size five by a foot, no pun intended.

Death is the great equalizer. As we struggled with who got what or loaded up the car with Mother's discards for the "Bibles for Missions Thrift Store," the question of earthly possessions gyrated. How sudden the descent of treasure into trash. We would comment about something we were doing, especially as we shed more things, "Mother would hate this." I refuted those doubts with "she sees our hearts now." Her Memphis persona would no longer judge us.

We spread her life's treasures on the table, on cabinet tops, and across the floor. We set out platters, tarnished serving dishes, china, crystal, a silver coffee service, wooden candlesticks made by Daddy, ceramics created by Mother, quilts, art painted by Aint E and Mother's friends, lamps, oh yeah, tables, beds, chairs, several sets of flatware. Plus the kitchen of a consummate cook. All to be dispensed with the clock ticking for family members to get back to work and normalcy.

The divisions did not go as smoothly as we hoped. We made piles, loaded up boxes, taped and labeled the boxes to be hauled on long trips in trailers, by movers and even in the U.S. mail. We stashed the boxes in closets at Mother's until that journey.

We found her stockpile of yardsticks in her sewing closet along with expensive scissors and pinking shears. We knew the yardsticks from our childhoods. We recognized the thick one used for punishments, the lighter one to measure a ream of fabric. Other stories surfaced, Mother with switches in the backyard, when we sat on the swings crying, the skin of our little legs broken by the switches. No wonder we did not think some of Mother's Alzheimer's behavior aberrant.

One last day together: we fought, cried and compromised, parading out ancient slights and childhood dynamics. We had barely made a dent in the physical remains of Mother's life. But we all said goodbye, love you, peeling away sister by sister.

And then there was only me, overwhelmed by the work ahead. I lived alone in Mother's home for three months, sleeping on the antique bed in the guest bedroom, waking up to a ghost world populated by her memories. Each day I got up, had my green tea, and scavenged through her life. My sisters came as often as possible to facilitate the unraveling of Mother's braided holdings, but mostly it was a solitary undertaking. I rummaged through closets and drawers, making finite decisions in days that dragged on like a stalled infinity.

Everyday I cleared out her belongings; some earthly possessions transferred into full garbage cans, others made accessible for sisterly assignments. Drawers and closets were emptied, all brought out into the open, into an unknown future. Mother's mental anguish became evident as I picked through the scraps strewn throughout her home. I found notes she wrote: in baskets, notes in the kitchen, in bedside table drawers. Notes in her tight handwriting to remind herself of her name and other pertinent information, prompts about where she lived or why she was calling.

Frightened by the spillage from every crevice, I would get stuck in a hospital recollection, hearing Mother's childlike demands, her face gaunt, her fists pounding, "Mine! Mine! My play pretties!" The image transported me back to ancient Mississippi vocabularies, to country folks who stared grimly back at me from photo albums. Thoughts ricocheted between useless EEGs and handwritten recipes, between risky Abilify and church bulletins mimeographed with the Sunday morning scripture reading from 1958.

Opening all the blinds in Mother's home, I desired to let in the light, to dispel the shadows. In the hospital, during her all-night freak-outs, she would ask, "Are the doors locked?" The loop of concerns, "Are the blinds closed?" After saying yes, I would walk across the hospital room and pretend to close the shades of her hallucinations. Though intensified during those lonely hospital nights, Mother had always been afraid that danger lurked right outside of her closed blinds, that someone might look inside through the open curtains and comprehend our vulnerabilities.

My sisters preferred less looking through everything and more chucking of the morass of papers: let bygones be bygones. I, on the other hand, searched for my mother before she lost her mind. Here was my last chance to unknot the enigma.

Mother kept every thank you card she ever received: for dinners, luncheons, birthday parties, for teaching an inspirational Sunday school class. I discovered cards and letters from us, her daughters, from her grandchildren, Mama Mat, Elois, people I didn't know, and best of all, Daddy. Intertwined were meaningless church phone directories, yellowing newspaper articles and Walls' Automotive newspaper ads. She had kept Papa Vinson's tax forms from the 1930s and loan receipts from his neighbors who purchased essentials at his store, pencil scratchings of fates long forgotten, harvests promised, droughts' interference. I kept digging, the overflowing trashcan beside me, and excavated the car title and annuity statements, unearthed checks Daddy had written in the 1940s. "Don't even think about why she saved those checks," I thought, my hands dusty with the past.

Mother had secreted away her life before babies. The loveliest revelations emerged from far in the back of her closet, from a box with big hand-written letters: "HOWARD." Underneath a lifetime of birthday, get well and finally sympathy cards for his death, beneath the Shriners fez and Highland Street photos, lay Mother's love letters to Daddy. (Did she find them in his hidden treasures after he died?) In a more rounded handwriting, on lined paper, she teased, vamped and entertained for him, always with cajoles to come down to Blue Springs soon. These romantic missives ended with an underlined "I love you so much." From Mississippi indolence into Howard's work world in Memphis she wrote to him. "I never imagined anyone would be so kind and good to me."

Judy carried a top-heavy mound toward the back door and the big aluminum garbage can by the gray wooden fence. "I think this is all junk, but do you want to look?" In Memphis for the weekend, Judy was wearing Capri pants in the springtime warmth.

"Sure," I agreed, knowing how the unexpected had turned up in unaccountable places. I rubbed my dirty palms on my blue jeans.

Judy dumped everything on the kitchen cabinet, and we casually shuffled through the top layer. "What's this?" Judy wondered when she came upon a thin, square box, covered in gold textured foil. We opened the lid with the worn edges of fanned cardboard to find Army insignia. They did not belong to Daddy; he was deaf in one ear and hard of hearing in the other, and in spite of a night train from Memphis to Georgia, the army twice rejected him as 4F and sent him back to less heroic endeavors. I fingered the Purple Heart, the sergeant's bar and a blue replica of a 1800s rifle surrounded by a silver wreath. From attic treasures, saved newspaper articles, pictures and conversations I created my vision of Willie Lou and Thomas.

MISSISSIPPI PAST

Willie Lou and Thomas met as kids living in Guntown, a diminutive spot without a main drag or sidewalks: only quiet dirt roads and hardscrabble farms. Willie Lou and Thomas were high school sweethearts, both with a straight part in neatly combed and flattened hair, learning those delicate lessons of first love at Cedar Hill School. There were ten rural Mississippi teen-agers in their 1938 senior class. In modern parlance Willie Lou and Thomas were the Cedar Hill High School power couple. Willie Lou was senior class president and Thomas was vice-president. She played on the girls' basketball squad, he on the boys. He was the assistant editor of the fledgling school newspaper; she was the news editor. She was also editor of their school yearbook, The Pioneer, its loose leafed pages book-ended by stiff black paper covers, the uniformly-rectangular photographs individually hand-glued into each yearbook. In those innocent days their 1938 class motto was, "The world is a mirror, smile at it and it smiles back at you."

After graduation, Willie Lou went to Blue Mountain College, a protective Baptist girls' school, a little distance north on paved highway 15. Again she played on the basketball team. She made good grades but argued with her roommates, especially during all night study sessions. Though she was in love with Thomas, she sometimes dated other boys, several of them wanting to marry her, which seemed to be more commitment than could be said for Thomas.

Thomas went to work for a drug store in Batesville, a short drive to the west of Guntown. It seemed a natural progression for

Thomas since in high school he had worked at the small store in nearby Blair, Mississippi owned by Willie Lou's father, Papa Vinson. Besides, the Cedar Hill senior high prophecy had predicted: "Thomas is running a store all by himself. Fancy that! He is looking forward to the next J.P. election. He specializes in selling school kids mechanical pencils that make no mistakes." Everyone expected Thomas to do well for himself, particularly Willie Lou. She adored him.

Willie Lou and Thomas continued their relationship, as saved photos revealed. In those sepia secrets, darkening with time like dusk across a cotton field, Willie Lou appeared playful and amused, decked out in big fake pearls, a wide belt cinching her nubile body, her hair pulled back from her fresh face with a bobby pin. She was looking up at Thomas, who wore a coat and tie. Holding his hand, Willie Lou grinned, there beneath the bare tree branches.

Stories of war and gory atrocities in foreign countries were making their way into American newspapers; startling headlines set in large type, even invading local gazettes delivered weekly to mailboxes along tranquil rural routes. The world did not smile back, in spite of yearbook dreams, and in January 1941 Thomas joined the Mississippi Rifles, a National Guard Unit. What Mississippi native son wouldn't be proud to be in the 155th, which got its start fighting under Jefferson Davis and Andrew Jackson? Those who joined the National Guard early in 1941 were assured that after a year of training they would be released and not drafted. Just about the time Thomas and the Mississippi Rifles were set to go home for extended Christmas furloughs, their duty nearly complete, the Japanese bombed Pearl Harbor, pummeling pleasant high school promises. Young men lost the privilege of running their own stores, and neither mechanical pencils nor blood could stop the terror ahead.

Thomas went into the Army, and Lou taught school after her college graduation. The world was in turmoil. Elois had married Jack, a smart, happy-go-lucky fellow, and she moved around to various bases with him during his Army trainings. Elois found jobs wherever they went, as the country exploded into a war machine.

Thomas' regiment started at Fort Blanding, Florida to guard the Atlantic coast against feared invasions. It took years to train the troops and get enough equipment to fight the enemies overseas. The 155th became a training battalion, carrying out maneuvers in Florida, Louisiana and Texas, readying other troops to ship out. Thomas sent Willie Lou pictures of himself in front of hastily built barracks and in pith helmets left over from World War I. She saved those pictures along with the letters, the valentine cards signed "I love you" and a book of poetry. She was an English major and actually liked reading poems. She called him her fiancé.

In 1944 Jack finished OCS and shipped out for the European theater. Thomas and the 155th left for the Pacific. Elois and Willie Lou moved to Memphis to work at Kennedy Hospital, newly built to care for wounded soldiers. It had been many years, but the sisters were again sharing a room, this time in their cousin Glady's house.

Willie Lou's moods roller-coastered in response to her letters from Thomas. Like a whole world of women missing their men, Willie Lou spent hours writing to Thomas, living in the words in her brain, yearning to hear from him, distressed about the war. One Sunday, reeling after an especially disappointing letter from Thomas, Willie Lou stayed in bed until the middle of the afternoon while her cousin Glady's family shared lunch. Elois wrote to Jack about her sister's moping, but my mother, the consummate worrywart, had grist to the mill for her fears. On the front section of the *Commercial Appeal*, the bold headlines of May 15, 1945 announced, "Bloody victories at Mindanao exact Midsouth Toll." That newspaper wore a patina from Lou's nervous fingers, because Thomas's division exacted both victories and losses in that bloody fight for the Philippines.

The Mississippi Riflemen, along with other southern boys, were taking back the Philippines, making good on MacArthur's promise to return. They had once again earned their name, the Walking 155th, by battling their way along Sayre road, where the Japanese had dug in and were fighting to the death. Their path through other Pacific islands had taught the Dixie unit about fighting in the jungle. They knew the tropical thickness, its sounds more intense than southern swamps; knew that tree roots, snakes, dysentery and rain could down an infantryman as fast as bullets. These men, boys really, had assaulted foreign islands, knee deep in white-capped waves and loaded with packs and equipment; had advanced through the ear-splitting reign of mortar fire and screams of despair; had stuck cigarettes in their noses against the smell of decaying flesh. They were doing it again in the Philippines.

In June 1945 Mama Mat and Willie Lou were sitting on the porch in Blue Springs, hand stitching. Apprehension, like inlaid wood, textured the quiet air. Talk was always of the war, concern about the boys, the battles dragging on. Of course they had fretted about Jack. He had been wounded in France. Although Jack wrote home that he got a little nick on his leg, he almost bled to death from a shrapnel explosion. He was nearly captured at the evacuation hospital near the Battle of the Bulge. For many months they had no idea where Jack was or how he was doing. In April he was finally brought to Kennedy Hospital, where Lou and Elois worked, to recover. He was in a full body cast and no one knew if he would walk again.

June in Mississippi languished on the humid edge of hot. The Nazi regime had surrendered. Fighting had ended in Europe in May, but the fighting continued in the Pacific theater, especially for Thomas's Dixie Division.

Mama Mat sat on the front porch swing, as she finished sewing on the last button, securing the thread and biting it off with her teeth. She probably held the blouse up to check out her handiwork. The chickens were scratching and clucking behind the house, the cows grazed in the pasture beyond the barbed wire fence. No letters had come from Thomas in weeks. The slowness of mail from the front lines kept fates hidden. For quite a while Elois didn't even know Jack had been wounded. None of that comforted Willie Lou as she pulled her skirt around her bare legs.

Papa Vinson's mother, Ma Robbins, was living with Mama Mat and Papa and would die in their house in the next month. Perhaps Willie Lou went inside to check on her grandmother and the screen door slammed shut behind, a loud slap disturbing the calm afternoon on the farm. A truck heading up the road left a tail of dust as it turned onto the wide Vinson yard, driving up close to the house. It was Mr. Brown, Thomas's father, and Annie Maude, the wife of Thomas's big brother. Willie Lou depended on Annie Maude as her high school Home Ec teacher, later as a neighbor and friend. In Willie Lou's plans she and Annie Maude became sisters-in-law. I can imagine my mother standing on the steps of the concrete porch anxious for them to have good news about Thomas.

Thomas, a southern country boy stuck behind an embankment for days, was killed at the very end of the war, in May of

1945. He got a Bronze star posthumously; he and five others in the mortar section held their position, as the newspaper article praised, "through a concentration of Jap fire."

The U.S. took the island, atom bombs were dropped on Japan and VJ Day came in August, only three months after Thomas was killed.

Mother never told me how deeply Thomas's death affected her, though it lived as a dark secret of her past. Her whole life Mother's emotions got the better of her. She cried at the drop of a hat and she often succumbed to sick headaches. No doubt she went crazy with grief after Thomas was killed, her dreams of marrying him destroyed in a foreign jungle. Likely Mother's Mississippi community who had spoiled her as a child, rallied to comfort her as the war took away her innocent dreams. As teen-agers my sisters and I found a treasure trove in the attic, a box of letters written on thin airmail paper from Willie Lou to Thomas when he was in the Dixie Division. Certainly we gave them a quick read before taking them downstairs to ask our mother about those love letters. She took the letters, chagrined, and later trashed them. She must have felt disloyal to Daddy when our girlhood nosiness found those letters, though toward the end of her life she admitted regret at not preserving that piece of history. A reflection of war widows, Mother sought the forward momentum that drove the world to continue after such massive grief. Mother went back to work at Kennedy Hospital and celebrated with Elois when Jack took his first halting steps with crutches.

Mama Mat wrote to her daughter during that time of sadness. The writing was in ink, not the usual pencil, on lined notebook paper from a small pad, beige with time. The letter required attention to decipher, complicated by a total lack of punctuation, misspellings, and shaky handwriting.

Dearest Willie Lou

your Dads in the field and we are done washing long ago.

We do hope all is well and Jack is not to tired from his trip we have waited a long time for that time and then it had to be so sad Willie Lou I don't know what to say only do the best you can try to eat and sleep some so your health wont give under this if you cant make it up there try coming home for a few day the more you think about it the worse it is to me I don't know how you feel but I do know it is just to sad to be so Just do the best you can for you are as dear to us as Thomas was to you and we loved <u>him</u> two but thay say God know best. We are all so worried about you and love you so much.

your Dad said a man with boys hadn't any worse times than we have jack wounded and Thomas gone.

so every body come home any time you want to and can

Please write us for we are all way so glad to here from you love for all Mother

<u>MEMPHIS, APRIL 2009</u>

It all became too much for me, the war wounds, the church recipe books, the Blue Mountain College diploma that meant so much to Mother but no one wanted. (One day when Mother was mad at all of us in the hospital she explained angrily, "Blue Mountain! Blue Mountain! Blue Mountain! Control! Control! Control!" Her education justified her commands.) For several days I let the telephone ring without answering it. Like I normally did at home. But it turned out to be an escape not allowed in Memphis. When I returned phone calls to my sisters a few days later, they were channeling Mother's fears. Judy thought I'd fallen from the attic when cleaning it out or that I had been taken at gunpoint by someone who was going to steal all of Mother's money from the bank. Bev was more convinced that I'd gotten drunk, hooked up with some stranger (what, is it the 70s again and I missed the time travel), and had a wreck. They actually told me this when I called them.

Grief can exasperate anxiety. What I needed was to withdraw and, metaphysically, lick my wounds. I was tired of crying, of facing Mother's finiteness every morning, while my sisters had work, husbands and kids to attend. I had Mother every waking minute. I no longer cried that she had died; that was truly a blessing. I cried in response to the sadness of watching her die, of looking at how she hoarded, of how her friends missed her.

The ancients had the "red tent" for menstruating women, where they got to escape and rest during their periods. I wished for a "blue tent" to grieve and recuperate, where the world outside would halt and take care of me, defending against further losses. Either modern life doesn't allow such indulgences and recoveries, or we don't know how to do such a thing. We move on and eventually the feelings of loss and change might express themselves in some insane voice, in a surprising emotion or absurd choice. I heard of an African grief ritual where villagers swirled emotionally around a fire for three days after the loss of a villager. Every one had to participate in this ceremony because it was believed that those who didn't grieve communally would become the village troublemakers the next year. Modern culture offered no such outlets, perhaps creating a village of troublemakers.

Each family deals with death and its remnants differently. I knew cousins and friends who closed up their parent's house, lipstick remaining on the dresser where their Mother left it before she was rushed to the hospital. Others jammed all their parents' personal effects into a storage unit for several years. It may be worth it to walk away and come back to the task unburdened. I might have done the same thing as an only child. My agenda was not exactly what the executor was bound to do, but I was mesmerized by the tiny details. My sisters had bigger goals for me. Clear out everything and sell the condo. They thought I was "dwelling" on the past and called to check on my progress, coming when they could. I was as quick as I could be with the throwaway switch, but in mourning everything reminded me of how little I knew, how much I'd missed about my Mother. Though I couldn't ask her anything, she left me clues everywhere. Because she never threw anything away. Nada.

Every Sunday in Memphis after Mother died I went to her church. The sun streaked through the red stained glass windows. I carried small boxes for Mother's church friends. I had found gifts they had given her, cards thanking her, shells from some Texas beach. I collected those things, along with photos of them together, maybe a scarf, wrapped them with ribbons from Mother's hall closet, a note from me thanking them for what they meant to Mother and to me, and placed it in their hands as the organ swelled. They cried, because their daily life would be more affected by her absence than my routine back in Seattle might be. I did the same for her granddaughters. I collected cards, photos, belts, or clothing and sent those boxes to them. Always I added a note to friends and nieces: "These small gifts are an expression of Lou's presence while you learn to live with her absence."

Chapter 17

DO THIS IN REMEMBRANCE OF ME

> *"We might, in that indeterminate period they call mourning, be in a submarine, silent on the ocean's bed, aware of the depth charges, now near and now far, buffeting us with recollections."*
>
> *Joan Didion,* The Year of Magical Thinking

Memphis, Spring 2009

Mother loved to keep newspaper articles, on Parkinson's because of Elois or wedding announcements from forty years ago. She clipped them from her daily *Commercial Appeal* or *Press Scimitar*, cutting clean edges and sharp angles with her good scissors, articles on Alzheimer's disease, more recipes. My vigilance in looking at all this outdated news was rewarded one spring day, as the sun blasted through the open windows. I found very tattered, yellowed articles from the Memphis newspapers about the bus fire. It was big news in Memphis in 1952. On the front page I read the capital letters, "11 Baptists Are Injured as Blast Rocks Chartered Bus."

THE BUS FIRE

I was five the summer of 1952. Mother and Daddy chaperoned a busload of Memphis church people, a yellow transport of mostly fresh youthful faces from Prescott Memorial Southern Baptist Church. They were traveling together under the religious dome of "young people" to the Baptist assembly just east of Ashville, North Carolina. I probably wanted to go with them. For even as a young child, I was aware of the importance of church to my family. We seemed to go to church all the time, and I recall being ensconced in love there. I was especially enamored with the "young people's department," a college-aged group that claimed Mother and Daddy as their leaders. College kids were lively, often funny, and heaped affection on me.

My parents' friends, Pete and Wileen, had been recruited to take care of my two younger sisters and me while my parents journeyed to the ether of the Baptist mountaintop. Pete and his wife Wileen temporarily moved into my family's small two-bedroom house bringing two little blond boys of their own. Besides Pete managing Daddy's "automotive parts and service," our families often spent time together: at birthday parties with munchkins high on homemade cake and presents, during lazy afternoons as our mothers got their hair cut in each other's living rooms, and for southern suppers. Wileen had a sweet face and thick, shiny hair. Pete, a kind man, had lost some fingers in a previous career as a butcher and must've found selling spark plugs for my dad easier work than meat carcasses and sharp knives.

My parents were supposed to be gone about two weeks. Modern interstates did not exist in 1952 to accommodate their long journey across the natural cathedrals of the southern Blue Ridge Mountains. I didn't mind. I was already charmed by Pete and Wileen's son, Mike. With Wileen's fair complexion and soft features Mike, at six-years-old, was an older man in my kindergarten world. Wileen had her hands full with a cascade of five children from first grade to first year. During those humid Memphis afternoons Wileen spread quilts over clotheslines to make tents for our games. Whatever we played bubbled purely from our imaginations. It would be a few years before Mike added kisses to our playtimes: Mike as a pretend ambulance driver, his sensual boy lips on my cheek as he rescued me. I nourished a crush on him that would color our friendship for decades to come. Much to my disappointment in high school, he became enamored with my sister Bev. Telling me about his yearning for her, he would sing the Lovin Spoonful song, "A younger girl keeps a-rollin' 'cross my mind, no matter how much I try I can't seem to leave her memory behind." Impatient for her to grow up, Mike wanted Bev to be the lucky recipient of his kisses. Still, his later infatuation with Bev did not diminish his permanent status as my first boyfriend, a romantic notion that flourished in 1952 when we were tanned children crowded into an 850 square-foot house.

Like my mother, Wileen had the help of our African-American maid, Nonie. Nonie cleaned and ironed, starching sheets and blouses, while listening to her "stories" on the Philco console radio. By 1952 the art deco Philco had been demoted from the living room to the dark hallway, after being usurped by our first television. Even after her radio soap operas materialized on the magical medium of television, Nonie still had to keep up with her "stories" from the voices on the Philco. A 16mm black-and-white home movie showed a grainy Nonie striding our tiny backyard. Tall and regal, she moved with graceful assurance, her uniform gray with a white apron. Nonie spoiled my sisters and me. In return we adored her. And that hot summer when I was five, Nonie, sweating over the ironing board close to the Philco, proffered another steadying influence in our makeshift household, a comforting fixture in an improvised family to shelter me until my parents returned.

After a few weeks, in the manner adults use to tempt children with a bribe from the future, Wileen promised, "Your mommy and daddy will be home tomorrow!" Offered like dessert if you clean your plate. "We'll go to the church in the afternoon and meet the bus when it gets here. They'll be so glad to see you!" She had just mothered five children under six years old for two weeks, and she might've been happier about the prospect of my parents' homecoming than I was.

However, Mother and Daddy didn't get home the next day. Wileen explained to us, "Your mom and dad won't be getting home today. The bus broke down and they have to get it fixed."

The only phone rang shrilly in the hallway of our diminutive post-war house. Wileen would rest the clunky black receiver between her ear and shoulder and go as far down the hall as the phone cord allowed. A small girl in ruffles I hid beside the tall and wide Philco radio trying to listen to Wileen's phone calls and hear more about Mother and Daddy.

Our Philco, a 1946 floor model radio and phonograph with decorative inlays, provided the perfect shadow for my lurking. At the time my parents married and brought their new electronic console upstairs to their first apartment, it reigned as "the Cadillac of radios." They were oddly alike, the Philco and my parents' marriage. Both sprang from the end of the war; both were swept up in the world's rush to normality.

Philco's trajectory reflected the American middle class in general and my parents in particular. The company built refrigerators, washers, dryers and radios until the early 1940s. Old movies featured families collected around a radio, chuckling to comedies like "Fibber McGee and Molly," gaining strength from FDR's "Fireside Chats" or alarmed to hear the static-filled announcement about

Pearl Harbor. In 1942 Philco left civilian desires behind and completely converted to the invisible wares of the war effort, to radar, fuses and quartz crystals. When new Philco radios reappeared in American homes in 1946, after the war, my parents' version originally cost $205, expensive compared to the minimum wage of forty cents an hour. Easy to imagine Daddy calling the Philco (with the fancy "tilt-front cabinet" holding the record player) "snazzy," as he unpacked his assemblage of vinyl records, swing music for future daddy-daughter dances.

As children we liked the Bakelite pushbuttons on the Philco. With our petite fingers we would pop them in and out, not caring about their real purpose of finding AM radio stations and short-wave signals. If I had understood short wave communications at that early age, I would have connected with those signals that curved around the surface of the earth and into remote regions. I would've followed those radio signals to the ends of the earth to find Mother and Daddy. Instead I eavesdropped on Wileen's hushed phone conversations. An air of secrecy filled the hallway, something more threatening than a broken-down bus. After all, Daddy was an expert at getting engines to run. He could surely get that bus problem resolved.

The phone continued ringing. Family and church friends asked for the latest update, commiserating about the delay with Wileen, her voice as soothing as the balm in Gilead, "healing for the wounds of God's people." Wileen's whispers and the Philco's silence did nothing to alleviate my girlish anxiety. Time smeared like finger paints in my little brain. Not even playing house with Mike eclipsed my bewilderment.

Each day Wilene amended her excuses. "They didn't get the bus fixed yet. They're looking for a part." Daddy had a parts department at "the place," why not get the part from there? "Maybe by tomorrow they can start back to Memphis. They'll be home soon." The next day Wileen retraced those words.

"How can it take so long to fix that bus?" I questioned. "Why don't they just get a different bus?"

"Well, that's a good idea. Let's write them a letter and say that." And Wileen sat us down with color crayons and paper to "write" to Mother and Daddy. My three-year-old sister Bev scribbled boldly on the notebook paper, while I drew stick figures holding hands in front of a box-like house. Wileen wrote in pencil for us, "We miss you."

The buttermilk days passed with aunts and cousins coming to entertain my sisters and me, to take us to the zoo, and to give Wileen a break. In spite of all the attention, the mystery of my parents' absence aggravated my kindergarten-sized worries. My unending presence beside the Philco, more haven than furniture to me, yielded neither enlightenment nor optimism. Finally the grown-ups told us kids a contoured version of the accident.

"11 Baptists Are Injured as Blast Rocks Chartered Bus." The newspaper with this headline had survived fifty-seven years in boxes moved from attic to closet as my parents' hard work provided nicer houses. It surprised me that their experience in the bus fire had gleaned such coverage in Memphis in 1952. However, cleaning out my mother's home after her death furnished substance to the vaporous impressions of my childhood. Tucked into the box with the newspaper accounts were those "letters" Wileen had helped us write, little girls' longings that I can only surmise Wileen saved to give to my parents. Then for fifty-seven years Mother conserved those drawings, our girlhood distillations of loneliness and art.

Some version of the bus fire resurfaced from time to time as a part of our family history. Daddy and Mother feared any flickers of heat near gasoline. If anyone smoked a cigarette close to one of his Esso gas pumps, Daddy, his voice usually steeped in horizontal southern vowels, would rush to the smoking offender and demand to have the cigarette snuffed out.

One vacation Daddy drove our family on the two-lane highways that snaked through the Great Smoky Mountain National Park. My sisters and I, probably teen-agers, sang and argued in the back seat. After ascending switchbacks into the darkened tunnels created by gray stone arches burrowed through mountain slopes, Daddy stopped in the parking lot at Newfound Gap. The wind blew cooler as we stepped out of the car and into the forests and clouds almost a mile up in the sky. We hugged ourselves against the chilly gusts. Newfound Gap was a notch between thickly wooded mountains, a scenic vista, and miles of jack-knife curves from any towns. Daddy stood beside a low stonewall, in plaid shorts with a cap covering his baldhead, and told us the terrifying details of their trip home from North Carolina in an ailing chartered bus.

"We stopped here for a prayer meeting at sunset, but the bus had already been having trouble. I went with the driver outside the bus to see what was happening. There had been smoke coming from the back of the bus." Ever the mechanic, that Daddy of mine, he would tackle any difficulty. Perhaps the old bus had simply overheated on the climb. Daddy and the driver bent down to see if there was a gas leak. "All of a sudden gas gushed out, it splashed everywhere." Daddy extracted his memories from that tremulous space, his slow syllables overpowering his typical reticence. "Then there was a loud explosion. People were on fire, some stuck in the bus and some outside. We started rolling anyone on fire down here."

We followed Daddy's eyes over the squat wall, down the slope of grass that halted at a stand of fir trees. Daddy's images came alive: getting those kids over the stone barrier, rolling them to put out the flames while chaos and screams surrounded him, the once-fragrant air rancid with smoke. "Then we'd stop cars that drove up here and get them to take folks to the nearest hospital. For a while we didn't know where everybody was, because some cars went up to Gatlinburg and some went south to Bryson City. The people who took those kids were mostly tourists up here to see the view." We listened to Daddy's calm drawl; listened transfixed where the bus had burned chaotically. Far from phone booths, doctors and hospitals, the safety of those Baptists from Memphis relinquished into the hands of strangers.

From those accounts I already knew Daddy had been a hero. But these newspapers I found, creased permanently by time in the back of Mother's closet, revealed yet another drama. "Plane Brings Home Heroine Who Saved Elderly Woman From Fiery Death." That heroine was my mother, Lou, whom the article described as a "pretty Memphis mother."

Traveling with the Prescott Baptist young people on their spiritual sojourn to North Carolina, a few other church members filled the remaining seats on the bus, including a 72-year-old woman, Mrs. Rhodes. The newspaper article continued with the recounting from a young woman on the bus. "Mrs. Rhodes had just stepped from the bus when gas that had somehow escaped, exploded and enveloped the bus. Mrs. Rhodes' clothes burst into flames, and she couldn't move. There was almost a wall of fire around her. Lou waded into the fire and pulled Mrs. Rhodes out, putting out the flames." My mother had literally saved a burning woman's life. The article ended with this tribute about my mother. "After it was all over, Lou kneeled in the road and prayed. I saw Lou's legs. What skin was left was in huge white blisters." Some young people surrendered into cars of strangers and my mother into the fiery hands of God.

As an adult I asked Mother about the bus fire. She told me without a hint of irony, "When Howard looked under the bus, he knew something was wrong. He came and told me get everybody singing. We started singing 'give me oil in my lamp keep me burning.' Your dad was wearing a seersucker shirt with yellow stripes. I can see it so plainly."

I read through the half dozen newspaper articles with ragged edges, humming the gospel song "give me oil in my lamp keep me burnin', keep me burnin' til the break of day." True to printed news delivered twice a day by a boy on a bicycle, all the articles were dated and filled with precise details. Over the years, just like the Philco, the newspaper clippings and childishly drawn family portrait had been shoved further back into a corner, only to be resurrected after both of the heroes had died.

Mother and Daddy came home, at last, on a propeller airplane. The bus had exploded, not broken down, the charred hulk beyond Daddy's magic. It had seemed like forever waiting for Mother and Daddy to return: a whole season of needing to understand what had happened, an infinity wondering when I would see them again. In reality, though, the interim had not been months. Mother and Daddy arrived back in Memphis only a week later than planned.

Daddy met us at the airport by a big wire gate and took us out on the tarmac, holding hands with Bev and me. Wileen, her own two boys in tow, carried my baby sister Judy. Beside the stilled airplane Mother lay on a stretcher before going to a Memphis hospital. Daddy, his face scorched and bandaged, hugged us tightly.

Daddy was grinning, and Mother was crying. There must have been a moment, the breath of a falling cinder, up in the seared atmosphere of the Smoky Mountains when Mother and Daddy thought they might never see my sisters and me again.

With their insurance money Daddy bought a 8mm camera and projector, and Mother bought a piano. They were planning a future for my sisters and me, putting the bus fire behind them, along with war, radio and 33 1/3 records. The young people from Prescott Baptist, many of them survivors of the bus fire, congregated regularly in our living room for fellowship. They sang around the new upright piano, while passing me from one hug to another.

Of course Mother raised my sisters and me with an overly protective agenda, predictable from a woman who once waded into a wall of fire. Ours was a controlled existence. Thanks to Nonie our bathrooms always smelled like Pine Sol and our floors sparkled. Nonie greeted us as we came in the front door after school. She hung up our coats, made us chocolate milk and cinnamon toast, all the while talking and listening. By the time I was in high school, the civil rights marches turned ugly and whites dug in. Nonie simply didn't come to work one day. She left a note for my mother, "I cant work for you no more." She most likely waited many years for the courage to speak her truth to Mother. Sadly, Mother and Nonie became a microcosm of the power struggle of the 1960s, collateral damage in a reconfiguration of conflict and normalcy.

Another casualty of those radical times: Philco filed for bankruptcy in 1960, their radio tubes antiquated like my mother's neurotransmitters. The company was bought by Ford Motor Company; their radios mobilized in Ford cars. As a child I had glommed onto the walnut console so intensely that as an adult I restored the Philco back to its rightful position in a bustling orbit. I moved it to the living room in my West Coast home. Then I fatefully filled its renovated interior with last century's CDs: the Philco destined forever to be a whimsical relic.

Mother and Daddy taught my sisters and me to kneel nightly beside our beds with folded fingers, praying our vulnerable souls into the benevolent Hands of the Almighty. Meanwhile Mother and Daddy and the other Prescott Baptist folks fearlessly sang at church gatherings, "Give me oil in my lamp keep me burning" because the eerie song ended with a rousing "Sing hosanna! Sing hosanna!" Prescott Baptist did love an inspiring hallelujah chorus!

Mother and Daddy remained friends with Pete and Wileen, eventually communicating from separate towns via long-distance phone calls and road trips in the RV. Cancer or Alzheimers stopped time for them. Without our parents, the kids pretending under the shade of a quilt in 1952 gradually lost touch with each other. But no matter how much I tried I can't seem to escape the memories of Mike's evanescent kisses, Wileen's tenderness, Daddy's seersucker shirt burned to a crisp, and my mother on her knees to the Lord.

Memphis, April 2009

I channeled Daddy in the brightly lit jewelry store. I wanted no more conflict between my sisters and me, wanted the disagreements about who got what finished, just wanted it all to rest in peace. In the store exquisite rings and necklaces sparkled in squeaky-clean glass cases, as I laid out Mother's jewelry, a feeble collection in the surrounding grandeur. But then Mother had never been one to indulge in shiny objects unless it was a new kitchen appliance. When Daddy really wanted to please her, he bought her a new sewing machine. Still, there were three cameos and three diamond rings, a Krugerrand necklace and other assorted pieces. Gold had reached all-time highs, and I was there to get appraisals on some jewelry and sell the rest.

Disappointment was instantaneous: the Krugerrand was fake, two rings were zirconium. I could foresee the fights about who would get the only real diamond ring, even though we had an accounting ledger to keep the distribution equal. In an exhausted state, I sold the one real ring with the other jewelry, putting over $600 in my pocket to distribute. Later that night I called my sister Bev, excited about the transactions.

"You sold the ring?" she gasped.

I was sitting in the high-backed blue velvet chair, talking into my pink cell phone. "Yeah, it seemed the best thing to do. It really wasn't worth that much."

"It was Mother's wedding ring!" she exclaimed.

I paused, reality hitting with the power of the big bang. "But she'd had it reset. It wasn't the original. The diamond was tiny."

"But someone would have wanted it!"

I got off the phone in a hurry to sink into a long night of berating myself, beating myself up for such a stupid mistake, and chastising myself for letting my sisters down. About dawn I crawled out of my sleepless bed and continued my internal diatribe. I started to cry. I imagined Daddy picking out the ring, wondered if he and Mother had chosen it together. I cried even more realizing I had never heard the story of how they got engaged. Big sobs. Shoulders shaking. Was Mother proud of her little ring, showing it off? What was she wearing? How did Daddy save the money from his fledging business? The only tidbit she gave us about dating Daddy was that "He always fell asleep on our dates. I almost didn't marry him." I was wailing by then, my face red and swollen, my nose snotty, a total mess crushed like a trailer park in a tornado.

Having survived all the ordeals of hospital, hospice, funeral, and the months dismantling Mother's home, and then, looking for the easy way out, I had sold her damn wedding ring. Me, the most sentimental sister, ditching the ring to avoid conflict. Bev was upset, and I couldn't imagine what Judy would say. I wiped my eyes on my sleeve, caught up in the hysterics known to southern women, all grounding washed away as in a Mississippi river flood.

Finally that night I called Bev back, barely able to talk, my voice garbled with tears. "I'm so sorry."

"I knew you were trying to do too much," she said in a dismissive tone.

I sniveled, laying on the peach love seat. "I'm really sorry."

"Well, just go to the store in the morning and see if you can buy it back."

I blubbered, "But there were so many people in the store selling their gold. It's probably already melted down."

"Just call," she suggested more kindly. Her practical notion comforted me and she soothed me with one of her own secret mistakes involving a wedding band.

The next morning I drank green tea waiting for the hour the store would open. After I told my story to the nice woman on the phone, she promised, "I'll look. But there's hundreds of pieces we've bought in the last few days." I imagined a pile of tangled jewelry, lambs to the slaughter, but gave her my phone number.

Then she called me, Mother's little ring in her hand. I rushed to the store to buy it back.

She sweetly refused the $20 tip I offered, explaining, "It happens all the time. You wouldn't believe how many times people change their minds."

I slipped the ring on my finger. There would be no arguments about the ring. It was mine. I had paid for it with twenty-four hours of craziness.

My sisters came for the final dividing, for shipping out the disputed marble-top table, and for packing up the last bits of our parents' life. Then Søren arrived to a condominium with empty rooms and random unwanted furniture. He and I drove to Cincinnati, heading east and north, pulling the trailer with the loot from his grandparents. It had been an unusually flawless spring in Memphis, azaleas and dogwoods redolent after the nourishment of extra rain.

"Just watch," Søren advised as we left Memphis. "Spring hasn't bloomed yet, further north."

Sure enough we appeared to be going backward in time, the buds tighter, unopened, the greens pale compared with the neons of Memphis spring. We traveled on into bare branches, from full blossoms into only the foreshadowing of flowers. I longed to carry Mother's belongings even further back into time: past the wet season, beyond the freak snow when we buried her. We would recede into some yesterday and set up her life again. In safe surroundings made familial by things she cherished, she could remember and she would spill her secrets.

Piles of mail on my table in Seattle awaited my return. Separating the junk from the important, I found a small box addressed to me in my mother's trembling handwriting. She must have mailed it right before she had the stroke. I tore the outer paper off the box, took scissors to the cardboard and pulled out a layer of bubble wrap, tightly taped. More scissoring, more layers of wrapping. A brown paper bag was uncovered, then a smaller, lighter box. "This must be something either very fragile or very precious," I thought as I un-mummified the contents. I didn't find it strange to be opening a package from my dead mother, even one obviously sent from the confines of a tortured mind. Neither did I think about her driving to the post office to mail this gift. Another layer was carefully cut away, only to reveal a swaddling of soft green fabric. Unfolding the cloth I found an inexpensive frame holding a picture of my grandmother and great grandmother.

What did it mean, the faded photo? Wide ribbons tied Mama Mat's dark pigtails, her hair surprisingly thick, and a white belt encircled her small waist. The puff sleeves of her white blouse were trimmed with the same lace as the narrow ribbon around her neck. Her jumper with big buttons down the front, I imagined as blue. She stood, her head tilted slightly, behind her mother, who had meant so much to my mother. Granny Susie, a petite woman, captured that long ago time, with her white hair pulled back plainly from her face. She had wire-rimmed glasses and a dress with a big round lace collar. Both ancient mothers wore unreadable gazes, the mysteries of their pain and joy concealed.

I imagined my floundering Mother in the last days of her life. She had enfolded layer upon layer of protection around the generations of motherhood, and from a kudzu'ed brain she entrusted the archive to me. It acquired a new home as a gray-toned presence atop the 1946 Philco in my living room.

Chapter 18

YOURS ALWAYS

"From the beginning/The end is in sight
Time is the rhythm/Love is the light"
The Last Song *by Robert Hunter and Mickey Hart*

Willie Lou was the baby of the Vinson family, the last girl of four born, and along with Elois, one of two who survived. Vassie Mae was three years old when she succumbed to a short life of illness. Mama Mat stood graveside in a loose black dress, roomy for Geraldine, the next baby growing inside her. Even in the uterus the allure of death must have caught in Geraldine's fibers, the darkness of the earth as sustaining as the wet womb. For Geraldine was born weak and spent much of her four years on this earth struggling for breath. By the time Geraldine died, Elois was seven years old. The soft voice Elois learned for not disturbing her feeble sisters became her meek timbre as an adult, a voice that still tiptoed past sick babies covered by a faded quilt of Mama Mat's careful stitches.

Since Willie Lou was just testing out the forward momentum of her fat baby legs, her ebullient nature was spared from seeing Geraldine's little white casket interred next to Vassie Mae. The elegiac rhythm --birth, birth, death, birth, birth, death -- echoed in the sad songs Mama Mat played on her guitar. Thankfully, the births had more verses, bestowing on Willie Lou the cadence to accompany a carefree child. She had a pet pig and dogs hanging out with her in the yard.

Eight-year-old Willie Lou, dark hair cut short over her ears, went down the road to a friend's house. After getting a drink of cold, sulfur-tasting water from the well outside, the two country girls skipped into the leaky house and sat down on the rough floor to play. Across the room the friend's mother cooked supper. The father stumbled through the door, crying. Willie Lou had never seen a grown-up man cry.

"We lost everything," he stuttered, catching his breath. "All our money. It's all gone. I went to the bank, but it was closed. We got nothin. How we gonna live without no money?"

Soon Mama Mat walked down the road. She wore a homemade dress, the farm wife's rural uniform from feeding the chickens at sunrise to serving suppertime leftovers to the pigs from a slop bucket. Charlie, Willie Lou's black and white dog, romped at Mama Mat's side, his tongue hanging from his wide doggie smile, dampening the dry ground with his panting slobber. The adults whispered with their backs to the girls, as Mama Mat tried to comfort her neighbors.

On the walk back home Willie Lou, frightened about what had happened, asked, "Did we lose all our money?"

Mama Mat explained. "Your pa drove to New Albany when he heard 'bout the banks closing. He said there was long lines of folks just standing round outside the bank, not knowin what t'do. Some of em crying even. He had our money in two different banks. So he hurried and went and got our money outta the other bank."

The financial frost of that day chilled the whole world, fear seeping into the cosmic psyche, including little Willie Lou. It was the Great Depression, and the Vinsons hung onto some of what they had. Sad men, desperate for work, would walk up and down the ruddy dirt road that passed the Vinson house. Those hungry men could always get something to eat there. Lou never forgot that desolation or those broken men. She became a frugal woman for the rest of her life, because she grew up when putting food on the table directed all daily chores. She blossomed into a woman who nourished others, a dedication which defined her.

The Vinsons moved around during Willie Lou's childhood as Papa Vinson looked for better ways to support his family. He taught in a one-room schoolhouse in Etta, Mississippi, where rot outlined the windows, highlighting hardship. Then another ten-mile move, improving his family's lot, eventually settling in Guntown.

Life changed little with these moves. Always in the farm communities the neighbor women gathered to make quilts, the cloth pieces hanging from the ceiling or on a big quilting contraption. Those hearty women, plainly dressed, would hand stitch and gossip, talking about what was going on along the hard-packed pathways, way off any main highway. The fabrics of Mama Mat's quilts were better than her poorer neighbors. The Vinsons sold fabric at their store, and Mama Mat took as much as she wanted from big bolts of fabric, suspended on the wall like colored steps of a textile ladder. The diminutive Mama Mat rolled the wide expanse of cotton material onto the wide counter, the long scissor blades noisy against the old wood. After the store was sold, Mama Mat used scraps from the clothes she sewed for her grandchildren on her Singer treadle machine. She made quilts with those left-overs: quilts she pieced together in wedding ring or butterfly patterns.

Like their mother, sewing became both a necessity and an art, the art of necessity, for Elois and Lou.

The Vinsons opened their home to relatives and friends. Their disparate collective lived together, fitting into small farmland houses. They shared the daily chores, weeded the garden, gathered the eggs, graduated from high school, all side by side. They sat around the table for every meal, a family sculpted by life's uncertainties. Beside the plates of fried foods and garden vegetables stood a jar of milk, the watery blue topped with a thick, rich cream.

After graduating from Blue Mountain College in 1941 Willie Lou taught elementary school in Auburn, Mississippi, where she boarded with a friend whose husband was away doing war work. Lou earned $62 a month and paid $20 each month for room and board. She next taught at Boyle in the Delta, where the blues were born organically out of that beleaguered life between the Mississippi and Yazoo rivers. The Delta housed the poorest of Mississippi poor, and Lou's pupils were no exception. They were a tough lot of kids, in their overalls and shirtsleeve tans. Although she had a hard time with some of them, she would one day show her teen-aged daughters stamp-sized sepia school pictures of those students, acknowledging that this boy or the other was "a handful." Lou lived in the "teacherage" with other young women like herself: room and board subtracted from her <u>annual</u> salary of $941. The students called her "teacher" and most weekends she took a rattling bus back to her parents' house in Ellistown. The bus route went from Cleveland, Mississippi north to Memphis, then south again to Tupelo, Mississippi, where Mama Mat and Papa Vinson drove over 25 miles to collect her. Once on the bus ride, when she was mad at

Thomas for not giving her a ring, she met a young preacher, whom she dated.

From the bus stop in Cleveland, Mississippi, Willie Lou had to walk to the "teacherage" in Boyle. If she could find a cab at her dawn arrival, she would take it; but more often than not she walked toting her suitcase at 5 a.m. through neighborhoods just beginning to stretch their muscles in the pink of sunrise. She was fearless in those days. Sometimes a kind bus driver would take pity on her and alter the route, steering his lumbering bus the three extra miles from Cleveland to Boyle to spare her that walk. Papa Vinson and Mama Mat wanted Lou home; perhaps because of the hard times of the war or maybe they worried about their youngest in such a dire environment, walking through a black section of town at dawn. They lured her with the promise of a car. She gladly left the Delta's troubled kids and was soon teaching at her alma mater, Cedar Hill.

The dissonant chord of death in the birth-birth-death-birth-birth-death chant vibrated intensely with the war's increased speed. The whole planet suffered. Willie Lou and Elois moved to Memphis and lived with their cousin Gladys and her family, six of them in a bungalow. Both Elois and Lou worked at Kennedy Hospital with its rows of brick buildings to house the casualties of war on acres of once-wooded land.

Elois wrote Jack long letters about the decisions she made that had been a husband's purview before the war. The maintenance of cars daunted the sisters. Elois wrote to Jack: she had found a nice man named Walls, who was trustworthy, to fix her car. Lou followed Elois' recommendation and got her car's brakes serviced at H. H. Walls Esso Station at Southern and Highland. It cost her $10, and her future husband signed the small ticket stamped "paid." Jesse, an African American, did the work, and ultimately Lou would write Jesse's weekly paychecks, until Howard retired. When Jesse died, Howard spoke at his funeral, standing in front of a congregation in an African American church.

When Jack, on crutches, and Elois moved back to Mississippi, Willie Lou continued to work in Quarter Master at Kennedy Hospital and kept the rare and much-envied apartment on Carnes Street. She adjusted to the changes even though she didn't like the women roommates who replaced her sister. Then another cataclysmic shift: Thomas killed in the Philippines.

Decades later the war remained beyond Lou's telling. Historians attest that her generation, surviving the Great Depression and the War, suppressed the experiences and moved on, side-stepping the pain, unable to articulate the depths of those tragedies. Lou refused to watch any movies about World War II. By destroying her letters with Thomas, Lou further rubbed out the physical evidence of that dark time, burying those secrets in an unmarked grave.

After the horrors of World War II, those remaining prayed for the return of the birth stanza of the birth-birth-death poem. Lou was pretty and smart, and in a world short on eligible men, Lou and Howard started courting. Perhaps Lou had heeded the condolences of a friend who wrote in a letter after Thomas' death: "There is no consolation but we just have to get ahold of ourselves and continue to make a life for ourselves that can be useful and profitable." By September, four months after Lou was told that Thomas had been killed, Howard was courting her.

Soon Lou was writing love letters to Howard, in cursive full and rounded, like her rosy cheeks, the words shaped as if an imaginary ruler measured each line. She had left her job at Kennedy Hospital for the coveted role of future homemaker. Being a wife, rather than being promoted at Kennedy, had always been her heart's desire. For weeks she stayed at her parents' house in Blue Springs, indolently planning her wedding.

My dear Howard

How strange it seems to be away from you so long. According to the theory of most people, one week, less than a week, isn't very long, but for me to be away from you who is close to me, who almost thinks for me and knows my every change of mind, is like an eternity.

Today Mama and I were sitting here wishing aimlessly. Mostly feeling low watching the rain pour down outside. We wished this, that. Finally, Mama said, "Know what I really wish? For the rain to stop." Then says I, "know the one thing I wish? Wish I could see Howard."

It has rained most of the day here. At noon I went to bed to pass away the time. The things I've done have been of little importance. I copied pages and pages of recipes. Fed my pet pig and the dogs numerous times. Dress (with a bath etc) about three. Oh as usual I ironed a bit here and there and packed this and that.

You'll get this letter Saturday. Course now, sweets, I don't want to interfere with business but what's the chance of your getting down early Saturday night? You've worked hard all week. Listen I'll be home so don't spend your time in New Albany again either. (orders.) I'm going to call you Friday, but this is a warning –an invitation (well, I can't think of the word, but I mean begging) pleading to come down Sat. night early. You can stay with us, huh?

Baby, I love you with all my heart. Yours always, Lou

Lou sat by an open window under her parents' green roof, surrounded by open fields and spring pastures, dreaming about Howard. She spent hours on beautifully written descriptions of country life and asking about Howard's fledgling business in Memphis. There she was, the college graduate, the English major writing to a man who struggled with the written word, a man who claimed "8th grade" on questions inquiring about "education." For years, when she went back to Mississippi to rest and visit family, Lou addressed folded epistles of love to his work place on Highland, into his long hours at the station. Coaxing him to her peaceful Mississippi world of sewing, Colliers' Magazine mysteries, and babies.

My darlin' Howard,

After leaving three unsolved murders, I have much difficulty in settling down to a so-called 'love letter.' Meaning, darlin' in the two issues of Colliers I had, three good exciting murders were committed – with a note at the end of this week's chapter 'To be concluded next week.' Whew! Such luck! Now I have to wait until I get into town to at least get any more light on the situation.

I kept telling myself you were coming down today (tonight), but I keep remembering that you are busy there while I do nothing but think here. Dot and I teased around all afternoon about Howard coming down. Maybe it was because I had that feeling that if I didn't see you that I would just die. Gosh, I wanted to talk to you so badly, but no means to do so.

Dear Howard

If anyone had told me this time last year that I would have been so much in love with you and so thrilled over soon becoming Mrs. Walls, I would have never believed them. It still seems like a strange wonderful dream that I will soon awaken from to find that I had overeaten – or something. Really, darling, I never even built an air castle high enough or big enough to hold such grand things as those that are happening to me now. Every girl wants to find someone who is as sweet and good as you, but few ever do. To think that I'm one of the very small percentage that has. What I'm trying to say, Honey, is that having you is one of the – no, the best thing that could ever happen to me. I love you – and thank you, darling, for being yourself—which is all I ask. Yours always, Lou

In April 1946 Lou and Howard married at the Baptist church down the road from Mama Mat and Papa Vinson's house. Mostly family attended, the women wearing suits and hats, the men handsome in their Sunday finest. Mama Mat and Lou did the flower arrangements, while a young Aunt Lottye was in charge of pictures, since she worked for a local photography studio. Lou was 24 years old and Howard was 33.

Lou's Mississippi roots were stretched taunt. Like other transplants, she would leave her new home in Memphis for a visit to familial soil, while Howard worked long hours building a business.

"Absence makes the heart grow fonder" resulted from these regular trips to Mississippi to collect food from the garden, to visit with family and friends from Guntown High School, and to "loaf."

September 1946
Dearest Howard

This visit would be lovely if you were here with me. Went swimming yesterday. Water nice. Whew! I miss you, honey.

We washed the clothes this morning. I wish I had a washing machine and a line. It took no time at all. I started out to help but changed jobs about the middle of it. I arranged flowers and loafed. Later we rested, had lunch and rested again. Guess what I did in the afternoon? I made the cutest blanket. I crocheted the prettiest blue (for boy) edge on it. I finished it last night then started on the little dress. I'm still working on it. You will simply love them. I told E last night your eyes would just light up and you would just have the cutest smile.

Darling, I love you so much. I wonder if I'll be able to stay down until Sat without you. Miss you so much. Yours always, Lou

On March 15, 1947, about six in the morning, Howard went to open the Esso station. He drove the only car they had, just to take care of a few things before he took his already-in-labor wife to the hospital. Elois and Lou stayed at the small upstairs duplex, Lou's contractions so bad that she was gripping the doorframe. In what would become family humdrum, Howard didn't come home like he always promised with a voice both sincere and distracted, despite the numerous phone calls to the service station. By the time

Howard got back, Lou's contractions were extremely close. They left in such a panic that he forgot Lou's suitcase.

Like many other women, Lou often told the story of that first difficult delivery, crocheting an emotional I.O.U. into my birthright. "I practically had Marilyn in the reception area of the hospital! She was born before 9:30 that morning. I nearly died when she was born. I had to have blood transfusions."

As an adult, Mother sent me a birthday card. In her fluid cursive she wrote, "The day you were born, the elements rejoiced and it snowed. Your dad forgot the suitcase. While he went to get it, your were born. He missed the big moment. The important thing is that you came to live with us and brought us much joy. I love you."

April 14, 1947
My dear Howard,

I never dreamed that life could hold so much happiness for any person as it did for me. Also I couldn't imagine any person being as sweet and considerate as you are to me. I consider myself the luckiest person in the world to have such a wonderful husband as you. God has been good to us.

Marilyn is sleeping and doing fine this morning. She cried all the way home from E's. When we got home, she was simply starved. I thought she would never get full. After finishing one bottle she was ready for another one. She really did sleep after she gave up. So did I. Imagine, I slept until seven o'clock.

I can hardly wait to get home to try out my new machine. Oh, you've no idea how proud I am of it. You are just too too good to me. I wonder what I did to deserve it.

Marilyn says she surely misses you, Dad, talking to her. She just laughed this morning. Bye. Yours always, Lou

Lou had gotten the washing machine she had wished for in an earlier letter. Later, in response to "What kind of men did your girls marry?" Papa Vinson said that Howard was too good to Lou. Everyone admired Howard's generosity and patience, and Lou savored his unselfishness. After all, Lou learned at an early age the delights of being spoiled.

In June of 1949 Beverly Jane Walls came into the world. In July Elois and Jack's 16-month-old baby, Brock, contracted polio. Even though epidemic, the source of the disease remained a mystery, and victims were isolated. Jack and Elois experienced the trauma of leaving their terribly sick baby in a hospital in Vicksburg, Mississippi, 250 miles away. Elois wrote pleading letters to doctors and nurses, desperate to know how Brock was doing and when her little son might come home.

August 1949
My darling

Things are busy around here this morning, as usual. Mama and Marilyn are cooking dinner now.

Marilyn is the happiest thing I've ever seen. Maybe it is all the space she has. She goes to the store with Papa and never leaves his side. I asked her what to tell you, "Come to Mississippi to see us. I love you." She doesn't want to come home.

We sure have lots of company here. Jack and Elois came yesterday afternoon. I was glad to see them. Jack & E thought Brock was better. They found out from one of the nurses that

Brock was affected in his back, both hips & left leg. E says he can't sit up. They didn't get any information from the doctor. He said that it is too early to make predictions yet.

We got 11 jars of peaches. And oh they are so pretty. I'll take another bushel & so will Mama. They are the prettiest I've ever seen.

Marilyn says to tell Daddy that the little chicken loves her. We are looking forward to seeing you this week. Do come. Please. We want you to. Beverly is calling. Better see about her.

Elois had twin boys in 1950, and Judy was born to Lou and Howard in 1951, enlarging the Vinson clan. Family reunions, piano recitals, church, and Brock learning to walk again time-stamped the 1950s. Like his father after the war, crutches barely slowed Brock down. In jars with holes punched in the lid with an ice pick the cousins collected lightning bugs, fascinated by the staccato flickering of the trapped illuminations.

Following the Vinson tradition of commitment to education, all three of Lou's daughters went to college. Memphis State University was a short walk along a street smelling of boxwoods, but my sophomore year I moved into the Memphis State dormitory only a mile from the columned house. One night my sorority-sister roommate and I made an elaborate glittered scrapbook in a messy version of a college all-nighter. Both of us rushed out of the dorm, leaving in our wake unmade beds, empty coke bottles, glitter, glue, paper scraps, overflowing garbage cans and clothes thrown over chairs. Later that afternoon we returned to a spotless dorm room. The beds had been made, floor swept, books put back on the shelves, everything straightened and tidied. The room had not been that clean all semester. The story of Lou stopping by the dorm room to leave some food and, probably in horror, conquering the total chaos became fodder for decades of reunions. It took years for me to see Lou's act as valiant rather than intrusive; for like worry, cleaning was also Lou's language of love.

A shocking secret became loosened from the family vault in 1970. Judy, a senior in high school, had dinner at a restaurant with Lou and Howard. An old friend came by the table and made small talk. Or so it seemed until the woman asked Howard, "Now, is Marilyn Lou's child or is she from your first marriage?" This divorce or that Howard had been married before Lou had never been mentioned. Locked away completely. Startling conversations followed. Howard would not let Judy tell me, afraid that it would affect my pregnancy. The news, however, quickly unfurled between the sisters. Months later, after Søren's birth, I sat at the piano in Memphis, playing softly as others got ready for bed. Howard, usually in his pajamas and asleep, stayed on the living room sofa, listening to familiar piano chords.

When I stopped playing and shuffled through other sheet music, just as I expected, Howard said, "You know about the divorce, don't you?" He explained. "I didn't know how to tell you girls, but I knew The Lord would take care of it."

Howard, of course, felt shamed to be a divorced man and relieved that Papa Vinson and Mama Mat had accepted him when he asked to marry Lou. Though a juicy tidbit, it did not affect the deep affection between Howard and his daughters.

When Howard died in 1990, Lou made her way bravely, but life wasn't as fun without him. She lived eighteen years as his widow, strong but lonely for his endearing attentions. No pleading missives could entice him to her side, no "yours always" to conjure his appearance.

Although Lou was insecure in perverse ways, she was fearless in others. In the 1990s after Howard died, she lived alone in the dream house they had built on a half an acre of genteel city property. One sunny afternoon during her widowhood she moved the Buick from the carport onto the driveway to wash it. Howard had always taken care of the family cars. He had catered to his "girls" in every way possible, keeping the family cars washed, serviced, and filled with (then cheap) gas before returning the vehicles to the females who surrounded him.

In what had previously been her husband's duty, Lou the widow sprayed the water from the green hose onto her car that day, a sudsy sponge wiping away summer dust. She drove the clean car, a shiny badge of her accomplishments, back under the carport.

As she got out of her sparkling car, the cacophony of a ring of keys and pepper spray in her dainty hands, a strange car drove up the wide driveway. Sometimes this happened, someone wishing to turn around or one of our friends from high school, now grown and stopping to visit Lou. Lou shut the car door and faced the unknown man who took bold strides toward her. Menacingly, he told her to go into the house, the shape of a gun threatening from his jacket pocket. He stood close to her.

Quickly she reasoned the danger. "My husband is in the house. He won't like you coming inside." She didn't know what this man might do to her. This was the same brave woman who walked to the Teacherage at dawn when she was young, who stepped into fire to save a friend.

"We'll go in the house anyway," the stranger threatened.

Lou feared that being in the house alone with him might be the end of her; she pointed her pepper spray toward the man and dowsed him. The culprit staggered, covered his stinging eyes and stumbled toward his car. Lou hurried into the house, locked the door and called the police. The man managed to drive away, tires screaming as he escaped. In the next few weeks, horrible neighborhood scenes ensued: break-ins and a nanny and the kids taken hostage. Lou had not become a victim. Pepper spray and daring had rescued her. My sisters and I praised her courage and called her the new sheriff in town.

As Lou faltered with dementia, her daughters continued to write letters, even though it's doubtful that Lou could focus long enough to read. At least it gave her gratification for all those walks to the mailbox. We kept telling her we loved her, praying that she understood.

Lou believed she was at the end of her days. All her life she had feelings or premonitions. She tried to tell my sisters and me that she knew how she was going to die, and it wouldn't be much longer, either. We, though, were still trying to fix her. After all, she and Howard had taught us never to give up, determination an entrenched family skill set. Knowing that her life was almost finished, Lou needed to say something about her life, to write her obit or say good-bye. That was not something she wanted to leave in the hands of her daughters. She pushed through the blizzard in her brain, her words lost in the snowdrifts, until she dug up the 18-year-old tribute written about Howard. It spoke of the commitments she and Howard had enjoyed together. It explained their shared creed: "to those to whom much is given, much is required." With help she put it in the mail to everybody in her address book.

After the strokes Lou at last got back to her own home, her craving sated. Although in a hospital bed, she lay in a safe place. Lou had barely spoken for days when I welcomed Aunt Lottye Kaye and Jim into the room.

Lottye Kaye exclaimed. "Why, she's wearin the pajamas I made for her." I had dressed Mother in red nylon pajamas trimmed with dainty red lace. Lottye Kaye smiled. "Lou, hi. It's Lottye Kaye and Jim. How're ya feelin?"

Much to the delight of everyone in the room, Lou awoke and perked up, joining in a conversation with Lottye Kaye. When Lottye would smile and ask Lou something, Lou was able to make only a few words, struggling with the effort, then trail off with "j-ja-j-je-j." Then Lou would laugh gleefully. Laugh with a joy long absent from her life.

"I brought you yams," Lottye told her sister-in-law.

Lou exclaimed, " I LOVE jja-je-j-j-!" Her face was full of eagerness and she chuckled some more, so unlike the woman she had been in recent years. And very unlike the one practically comatose for weeks. The conversation went like that, questions or statements from Lottye Kaye, Lou with her scarcity of words, trailing off with j-ja-ja-j and getting the biggest kick out of it. Perhaps being alive did "seem like a strange and wonderful dream" that she had described in her love letters to Howard, the horrors of dementia simply "like overeating." Now she woke up tasting only happiness.

Lou looked at Lottye Kaye, and with a big grin on her aged face proclaimed, "HOWARD j-ja-je-j-!"

Lottye Kaye, thinking of her favorite brother, paused, then acknowledged, "Yes, Howard was a good guy." A hint of Mississippi hung in her voice.

Lou smiled in agreement, her laughter like tintinnabulation. When Lottye Kaye and Uncle Jim said good-bye and we love you, Lou practically crowed, "I LOVE ja-ja-j-ja-je." Few words managed to escape the kudzu wildly running through Lou's brain, but it seemed only to amuse her. No one realized that those words, "Howard" and "love" would be the last Lou spoke, laying final claim to an unlikely match truly made in heaven. During that visit Lou radiated the essence of affection and laughter, as some ethereal choir sang "birth." Those of us in the room shared her amazement, echoing, "We love you too!" We cheered the splendor of Lou's lifetime of caring for others and honored the moment as she glided on generations of prayers.

ACKNOWLEDGEMENTS

Taking this long to write a book creates an extensive list of patient and helpful people to thank. First, there were the tolerant friends and family who read the earliest pages, before I improved my writing craft and focused the narrative. I thought because I could occasionally write a good sentence, it would be a breeze to write a book. Boy, was I mistaken!

One excellent foundation in the learning process included writing classes with Tamara Avila Guirado. After those classes the connections with Priscilla and Susan continued. Both women are incredible writers. They read my confused chapters, and their advice made me a better writer. Susan stuck with me until the bittersweet end of this book, and her organizational skills are unmatched.

I'm grateful to the friends who understood the solitude needed to write a book: you unsung heroines know who you are! I'm especially thankful to book club. They indulged me in reading pages to them, while offering me the courage to dream big. Two of "our book club husbands," Ron and Dave, went the extra mile, reading excerpts, eagle-eying typos, proofing the final manuscript, and taking nachos, beer or margaritas as payment.

Special thanks to Eli, the thoughtful and talented former editor of The Sound Consumer, who gave me assignments, ideas, and published my work. Our boss Trudy also championed my articles.

Dr. Afia Menke was my science and medical editor, parsing words, demanding more thorough explanations, and reading my work to her husband Dan. They kept me going when the task seemed endless.

My sister Bev drew the beautiful kudzu on the cover, and Jovanna was my dream graphic designer. Her deadlines encouraged me when I was running on empty. In a serendipitous revelation, I found that Jovanna had once lived in Memphis.

Family is essential in writing a memoir. My cousin Brock supplied details and memories with an unexpected kindness from a man of such brilliant sarcasm. Needless to say, my sisters shared their experiences and feelings with me, bravely recounting the details of difficult times with Mother when I knew they'd rather not talk about it.

My son Søren Palmer is the real writer in the family, and I am so proud of his dedication to his work. He read my chapters over the years and then generously edited the complete manuscript. He offered suggestions tenderly, but he also believed in me enough to recommend the harder changes. He is my example and my heart's song.

REFERENCES

Chapter 2: The Science of a Thousand Subtractions

[1] Alzheimer's Disease Fact Sheet. National Institute of Health, National Institute on Aging. Retrieved from http://www.nia.nih.gov

[2] Mild Cognitive Impairment. Alzheimer's Society. Retrieved from www.alz.org

[3] Ibid.

[4] Ward, A., Tardiff, S., Dye, C., Arrighi, H.M. Rate of Conversion from Prodromal Alzheimer's Disease to Alzheimer's Dementia: A Systematic Review of the Literature. *Dementia Geriatric Cognitive Disorders Extra.* 2013 Jan-Dec; 3(1): 320-332.

[5] Shenk, D. *The Forgetting. Alzheimer's Portrait of an Epidemic.* NY: Doubleday 2001.

[6] Fotenos, A.F., Synder, A.Z., Girton, L.E., Morris, J.C., Buckner, R.L. Normative Estimates of Cross-Sectional and Longitudinal Brain Volume Decline In Aging and AD. *Neurology.* 2005, March; 64(6): 1032-1039.

[7] Stern, Y. Cognitive Reserve in Aging and Alzheimer's Disease. *Lancet Neurology.* 2012; 11(11): 1006-1012

[8] Ibid.

[9] Wilson, R.S. Cognitive Activity and the Cognitive Morbidity of Alzheimer Disease. *Neurology.* 2010, Sept 14; 74(11): 990-996.

[10] Ibid.

[11] Finch, B. "The True Story of Kudzu, the Vine That Never Truly Ate the South." *Smithsonian Magazine*. September 2015. Retrieved from www.smithsonian.com

[12] Purdy, Michael C. "Falls May Be Early Sign of Alzheimer's Disease." 2011, July 17; Retrieved from https://source.wustl.edu/2011/07/

[13] Armstrong, R.A. Alzheimer's Disease and the Eye. *Journal of Optometry*. 2009, July-September; 2(3).

[14] Klunk, W.E. et al. Imaging Brain Amyloid in Alzheimer's Disease with Pittsburg Compound-B. *Annals of Neurology*. 2004; 55(3): 306-19.

Chapter 5: The Science of Your Brain on Alzheimer's

[1] About Alzheimer's Disease: Alzheimer's Basics. National Institute on Aging, NIH. Retrieved from www.nia.nih.gov.

[2] Hampel, H., Burger, K., Teipel, S.J., Bokde, A.L., Zetterberg, H., Blennow, K. Core Candidate Neurochemical and Imaging Biomarkers of Alzheimer's Disease. *Alzheimer's and Dementia*. 2008, January; 4(1): 38-48.

[3] Phelps, E. Human Emotion and Memory: Interactions of the Amydala and Hippocampal Complex. *Current Opinion in Neurobiology*. 2004;14:198–202.

[4] Rand, S. *Review of Clinical and Functional Neuroscience*. Chapter 9 Limbic System. 2006. Retrieved from www.dartmouth.edu.

[5] Suzuki, S. Scientists Show Hippocampus's Role in Long Rem Memory. *Science Daily*. 2004, May 13.

[6] Kryukov, V.I. The Role of the Hippocampus in Long-Term Memory. *Journal of Integral Neuroscience*. 2008 March; 7(1): 117-184

[7] Burgess, N, Maguire, E., O'Keefe, J. The Human Hippocampus and Spatial and Episodic Memory. *Neuron*. 2002 August; 35(4): 625-641.

[8] Maguire, E.A., Woollett, K., Spiers, H.J. London Taxi Drivers and Bus Drivers: A Structural MRI and Neuropsychological Analysis. *Hippocampus*. 2006; 16 (12): 1091-1101.

[9] Phelps, *Current Opinion in Neurobiology.*

[10] Adolphs, R. What Does the Amygdala Contribute to Social Cognition? *Annals of the NY Academy of Sciences*. 2010, March; 1191(1): 42-61

[11] Ortner, M., Pasquini, L., Barat, M., Alexopoulos, P., Grimmer, T., Förster, S., Diehl-Schmid, J., Kurz, A., Förstl, H., Zimmer, K., Wohlschläger, A., Sorg, C., Peters, H. Progressively Disrupted Intrinsic Functional Connectivity of Basolateral Amygdala in Very Early Alzheimer's Disease. *Frontiers in Neurology.* 2016; 7: 132.

[12] Lee, J.H., Ryan, J., Andreescu, C., Aizenstein, H., Lim, H.K. Brainstem Morphological Change in Alzheimer's Disease. *Neuroreport.* 2015, May; 26 (7): 411-415.

[13] Khachiyants, N., Trinkle, D., Son, S.J., Kim, K.Y. Sundown Syndrome in Persons with Dementia: an Update. *Psychiatry Investigation.* 2011; 8(4): 275-287.

[14] Retrieved from www.alz.org/braintour

[15] Frontotemporal Disorders: Information for Patients, Families and Caregivers. Retrieved from www.nih.nia.gov.

[16] Ibid

[17] Retrieved from www.alz.og/braintour

[18] Barendregt, M., Dumoulin, S., Rokers, B. Impaired Velocity Processing Reveals an Agnosia for Motion in Depth. *Psychological Science.* 27(11): 1474-1485.

[19] Ilg, U.J. The role of areas MT and MST in coding of visual motion underlying the execution of smooth pursuit. *Vision Research*. 2008, September; 2062–2069.

[20] Krauzlis, Richard J. Fundamental Neuroscience (Fourth Edition). 2013. Larry Squire, Editor. Academic Press. MA.

[21] Jeneson, A., Squire, L. Working memory, long-term memory, and medial temporal lobe function. *Learning Memory*. 2012, January; 19(1): 15-25.

[22] Retrieved from www.nidcd.nih.gov/health/aphasia

[23] Boksa P. On the neurobiology of hallucinations. *Journal of Psychiatry and Neuroscience*. 2009, July; 34(4): 260–262.

[24] Acheson, A., Conover, J.C., Fandl, J.P., DeChiara, T.M., Russell, M., Thadani, A., Squinto, S.P., Yancopoulos, G.D., Lindsay, R.M. A BDNF autocrine loop in adult sensory neurons prevents cell death. *Nature*. 1995, March; 374 (6521): 450–3.

[25] John J. Ratey. SPARK: The Revolutionary New Science of Exercise and the Brain. 2008. Little, Brown and Company. NY.

[26] Huang, E.J., Reichardt, L.F. Neurotrophins: roles in neuronal development and function. *Annual Review of Neuroscience*. 2001; 24: 677–736.

[27] Yamada, K., Nabeshima, T. Brain-derived neurotrophic factor/TrkB signaling in memory processes. *Journal of Pharmacological Sciences*. 2003; 91(4): 267–70.

[28] American Committee for the Weizmann Institute of Science "Bright Future for Brain Research." Retrieved from www.weizmann-usa.org

Chapter 8: The Science of Trouble Makers in the Brain

[1] Iqbal, K. et al. Tau in Alzheimer Disease and Related Tauopathies. *Current Alzheimers Research*. 2010, December; 7(8): 656–664.

[2] Brain's 'Garbage Truck' May Hold Key to Treating Alzheimer's. Retrieved from www.urmc.edu/news.

[3] Cepelewicz, J. Antimicrobial Mechanism Gone Rogue May Play Role in Alzheimer's Disease. Scientific American. May 26, 2016.

[4] Kolata G. Could Alzheimer's Stem from Infections? It Makes Sense, Experts Say. New York Times. May 25, 2016.

[5] Serrano-Pozo, A., Frosch, M., Masliah, E., Hyman, B.T. Neuropathological Alterations in Alzheimer's Disease. *Cold Spring Harbor Perspectives in Medicine*. 2011, September; 1(1).

[6] Koukouli, F., Rooy, M., Masko, U. Early and Progressive Deficit of Neuronal Activity Patterns in a Model of Local Amyloid Pathology in Mouse Prefrontal Cortex. *Aging*. 2016, December: 8(12).

[7] Aizenstein, H. J., Nebes, R.D., Saxton, J.A., et al. Frequent Amyloid Deposition Without Cognitive Impariment Among the Elderly. *Archives of Neurology*. 2008; 65(11): 1509-1517.

[8] Retrieved from www.lpi.oregonstate.edu

[9] Human amyloid-beta acts as natural antibiotic in the brains of animal models. *Massachusetts General News*. May 25, 2016.

[10] The Physiology of Stress: Cortisol and the Hypothalamic-Pituitary-Adrenal Axis. *Dartmouth Undergraduate Journal of Science*. February 3, 2011.

[11] Whitworth, J.A., Williamson, P., Mangos, G., Kelly, J.J. Cardiovascular Consequences of Cortisol Excess. *Vascular Health and Risk Management*. 2005, December; 1(4): 291-299.

[12] McGaugh, J.L., Roozenaal, B. Role of Adrenal Stress Hormones in Forming Lasting Memories in the Brain. *Current Opinion in Neurobiology*. 2002, April; 12(2): 205-210.

[13] Kim, J.J., Diamond. D.M. The Stressed Hippocampus, Synaptic Plasticity and Lost Memories. *Nature Reviews Neuroscience*. June, 2002; 3: 453-462.

[14] Green, K.N., Billings, L.M., Roozendaal, B., McGaugh, J., Laerla, F. Glucocorticoids Increase Amyloid-Beta and Tau Pathology in a Mouse Model of Alzheimer's Disease. *Journal of Neuroscience*. 2006, August; 26(35): 9047-9058.

[15] Dong, H., Csermansky, J.G. Stress Hormones on Amyloid-Beta Protein and Plaque Deposition. *Journal of Alzheimer's Disease*. 2009, October; 18(2): 459-469.

[16] Wilson, R.S., Evans, D.A., Bienias, J.L., Mendes de Leon, C.F., Schneider,J.A., Bennett, D.A. Proneness to Psychological Distress Is Associated with Risk of Alzheimer's Disease. *Neurology*. 2003, December; 61(11): 1479-1485.

[17] Wilson, R.S., Schneider, J.A., Arnold, S.E., Bienias, J.L., Bennett, D.A. Conscientiousness and the incidence of Alzheimer's disease and mild cognitive impairment. *Archives of General Psychiatry*. 2007; 64:1204–1210.

[18] Ju, Y.E., Lucey, B.P., Holtzman, D.M. Sleep and Alzheimer disease pathology – a bidirectional relationship. *Nature Reviews Neurology*. 2014; 10(2):115–119.

[19] Lim, M.M., Gerstner, J.R., Holtzman, D. The Sleep-Wake Cycle and Alzheimer's Disease: What Do We Know? *Neurodegenerative Disorder Management*. 2014; 4(5): 351-362.

[20] Ooms, S., Overeem, S., Besse, K., Rikkert, M.O., Verbeek, M., Claassen, J.. Effect of 1 night of total sleep deprivation on cerebrospinal fluid beta-amyloid 42 in healthy middle-aged men: a randomized clinical trial. *JAMA Neurology*. 2014; 71(8): 971–977.

[21] Depression May Increase Chances of Getting Alzheimer's. July 2010. Retrieved from www.livescience.com.

[22] Herbert, J., Lucassen, P.J. Depression as a Risk for Alzheimer's disease: genens, steroids, cytokines and neurogenesis – what do

we need to know? *Frontiers in Neuroendocrinology*. 2016, April; 41:153-71

[23] Goldin, A., Beckman, J.A., Schmidt, A.M., Creager, M. Advanced Glycation End Products. *Circulation*. 2006; 114: 597-605.

[24] Ibid

[25] Sasaki, N., Fukatsu, R., Tsuzuki, K., et al. Advanced Glycation End Products in Alzheimer's Disease and Other Neurodegenerative Diseases. *American Journal of Pathology.* 1998, October; 153(4): 1149-1155.

[26] Uribarri, J., Woodruff, S., Goodman, S., Cai, W., Chen, X., Pyzik, R., Yong, A., Striker, G., Vlassara, H. Advanced Glycation End Products in Foods and a Practical Guide to Their Reduction in the Diet. *Journal of American Dietetic Association*. 2010, June; 110(6): 911-916.

[27] Ibid

[28] Kerti, L., Witte, A.V., Winkler, A., Grittner, U. Rujescu, D., Floel, A. Higher Glucose Level Associated with Lower Memory and Reduced Hippocampal Microstructure. *Neurology*. 2013, November; 81(20): 1746-52.

[29] Ibid

[30] Above-Normal Blood Sugar Linked to Dementia. Harvard Health Publications. August 2013.

[31] Retrieved from www.alz.org.

[32] Retrieved from www.alz.org.

[33] Retrieved from www.diabetes.org.

[34] Attwell, D., Buchman, A.M., Carpak, S., Lauritzen, M., MacVicar, B., Newman, E. Glial and Neuronal Control of Brain Blood Flow. *Nature*. 2010, November; 468(7321): 232-243.

[35] DeFelice, F.G., Lurenco, M.V., Ferreira, S.T. How Does Brain Insulin Resistance Develop in Alzheimer's Disease? *Alzheimer's & Dementia.* 2014, February; (1Suppl): 526-32.

[36] Dore, S., Kar, S., Quirion, R. Insulin-like Growth Factor I Protects and Rescues Hippocampal Neurons Against Beta-Amyloid and Human Amylin-Induces Toxicity. *Neurobiology.* 1997, April; 94: 4772-4777.

[37] Yu, L.Y., Pei, Y. Insulin Neuroprotection and the Mechanisms. *Chinese Medical Journal.* 2015, April; 128(7): 976-81.

[38] Xu,W., Caracciolo, B., Wang, H., Winblad, B., Backman, L., Qiu, C., Fratiglioni, L. Accelerated Progression from Mild Cognitive Impairment to Dementia in People with Diabetes. *Diabetes.* 2010, November; 59(11): 2028-2935.

[39] Retrieved from www.diabetes.org.

Chapter 10: The Science of Reducing the Risks

[1] Ngandu, T., Lehtisalo, J., Solomon, A., et al. A 2 Year Multidomain Intervention of Diet, Exercise, Cognitive Training and Vascular Risk Monitoring Versus Control to Prevent Cognitive Decline in At-Risk Elderly People (FINGER): A Randomised Controlled Trial." *The Lancet.* 2015, June; 385(9984): 2255-2263.

[2] Shakersain, B., et al. "Prudent Diet May Attenuate the Adverse Effects of Western Diet on Cognitive Decline." *Alzheimer's & Dementia.* February, 2016; 12(2): 100-109.

[3] Berti, V., Murray, J., Davies, M., Spector, N., et al. Nutrient Patterns and Brain Biomarkers of Alzheimer's Disease in Cognitively Normal Individuals. *Journal of Nutrition, Health and Aging.* 2015; 19(4): 413-423.

[4] Smyth, A. Healthy Eating and Reduced Risk of Cognitive Decline. *Neurology*. 2015, May. On-line version.

[5] Warnberg, J., Gomez-Martinez, S., Romeo, J., Diaz, L.E., Marcos, A. Nutrition, Inflammation and Cognitive Function. *Annals of the New York Academy of Sciences*. 2009, February. On-line version.

[6] Most Americans Are Eating Better. June 2016. Retrieved from www.healthcare.utah.edu.

[7] Inflammatory Dietary Pattern Linked to Depression Among Women. November 2013. Retrieved from www.hsph.harvard.edu.

[8] Maron, D.F. Mediterranean Eating Habits Prove Good for the Brain. *Scientific American*. September 2015.

[9] Retrieved from www.techtimes.com/articles/161325/20160527/new-alzheimers-disease-theory-infections-may-trigger-build-up-of-amyloid-plaques-in-the-brain

[12] Gkougkolou, P, Bohn,M. Advanced glycation end products. *Derma-to-Endocriniology*. 2012, July 1; 4(3): 259-270.

[13] Ibid

[14] Ortinau, L.C., Hoertel, H., Douglas, S., Leidy. H.J. Effects of high-protein vs. high-fat snacks on appetite control, satiety, and eating initiation in healthy women. *Nutrition Journal*. 2014; 13 (1): 97.

[15] Mandel, S.A., Amit, T., Weinreb, O., Youdin, M.B. Understanding the Broad-Spectrum Neuroprotective Action Profile of Green Tea Polyphenols in Aging and Neurodegenerative Diseases. *Journal of Alzheimer's Disease*, 2011; 25(2): 187-208.

[16] Kuriyana, S., et al. Green Tea Consumption and Cognitive Function: a Cross-Sectional Study from the Tsurugaya Project. *The American Journal of Clinical Nutrition*. Retrieved from ajcn.nutrition.org. 2006.

[18] Stefani, M., Rigacci, S. Protein Folding and Aggretation into Amyloid: The Interference by Natural Phenolic Compounds. *International Journal of Molecular Sciences.* 2013, June; 14(6): 12411-12457.

[19] O'Connor, A. What's in Your Green Tea?" *New York Times*. May 23, 2013.

[20] Oulhaj, A., Jernerén, F., Refsum, H., Smith, A.D., de Jager, C.A. Omega-3 Fatty Acid Status Enhances the Prevention of Cognitive Decline by B Vitamins in Mild Cognitive Impairment. *Journal of Alzheimer's Disease.* 2016, January 6; 50(2):547-57.

[21] Kronenberg, G., Colla, M., Endres, M. Folic Acid, Neurodgeneration and Neuropsychiatric Disease. *Current Molecular Medicine.* 2009; 9(3): 315-323.

[22] World's Healthiest Foods

[23] Vitamin B6 for Brain Health. Retrieved from www.drweil.com.

[24] Micronutrient Information Center. Choline. Linus Pauling Institute. Retrieved from www.lpi.oregonstate.edu.

[25] Ibid.

[26] Ibid.

[27] Durk, M. et al. 1α,25-Dihydroxyvitamin D3 Reduces Cerebral Amyloid-β Accumulation and Improves Cognition in Mouse Models of Alzheimer's Disease. *The Journal of Neuroscience.* 2014.

[28] Littlejohns, T.J., Henley, W., Lang, I.A., Annweiler, C., Beauchet, O., Chaves, P., Fried, L., Kestenbaum, B.R., Kuller, L.H., Langa, K.M., Oscar L. Lopez, O.L., Kos, K., Soni, M., Llewellyn, D.J. Vitamin D and the risk of dementia and Alzheimer disease. *Neurology*, 2014, August.

[29] Deans, E. Selenium and the Brain. Psychology Today. October 2011.

[30] Whanger, P.D. Selenium and the Brain: A Review. *Nutritional Neuroscience.* 2001; 4(2): 81-97.

[31] Bradbury, J. Docosahexaenoic Acid (DHA): An Ancient Nutrient for the Brain. *Nutrients.* 2011, May; 3(5): 529-554.

[32] Stangl, D., Turet, S. Impact of Diet on Adult Hippocampal Neurogenesis. *Genes & Nutrition.* 2009, December; 4(4): 271-282.

[33] Dyall, S.C. Long-Chain Omega-3 Fatty Acids and the Brain: A Review of the Independent and Shared Effects of EPA, DPA, and DHA. *Frontiers in Aging Neuroscience.* 2015; 7:52.

[34] Cole, G.M., Frautschy, S.A. DHA May Prevent Age-Related Dementia. *The Journal of Nutrition.* 2010, April; 140 (4): 869-874.

[35] Ibid

[36] Pottala, J.V., Yaffe, K., Robinson, J. G., Mark A. Espeland, PhD, Robert Wallace, MD, MSc, and William S. Harris, PhD. Higher RBC EPA + DHA Corresponds with Larger Total Brain and Hippocampal Volumes. *Neurology.* 2014, February; 82(5): 435-442.

[37] Retrieved from http://www.whfoods.com

[38] Retrieved from www.lpi.oregonstate.edu.

[39] Walls, M. The Air Was Tart with Ripe Blueberries: A Study of Blueberries as a Microcosm for Choosing Whole Food. September 2000.

[40] Hribar, U., Ulrih, N.P. The Metabolism of Anthocyanins. *Current Drug Metabolism.* 2014, January; 15(1): 3-13.

[41] Krikorian, R., Shidler, M.D., Nash, T.A., Kalt, W., Vinqvist-Tymchuk, M.R., Shukitt-Hale, B. Blueberry Supplementation Improves Memory in Older Adults. *Journal of Agricultural and Food Chemistry.* 2010, April; 58(7): 3996-4000.

[42] Yu, A. The Wrong Eating Habits Can Hurt Your Brain, Not Just Your Waistline. December 2016. Retrieved from www.npr.org.

[43] Belluck, P. Another Potential Benefit of Cutting Calories: Better Memory. *New York Times.* January 26, 2009.

[44] Stein, R. Gut Bacteria Might Guide the Workings of Our Minds. November 18, 2013. Retrieved from www.npr.org.

[45] Ibid

[46] Robinson, M. Lila. New York: Picador. 2014.

[47] Bezerra de Pontes, A.L., Engelberth, R.C.G., Nascimento, Jr., E., Cavalcante, J.C., de Oliveira Costa, M.S., Pinato, L., Barbosa de Toledo, C.A., de Souza Cavalcante, J. Serotonin and Circadian Rhythms. *Psychology and Neuroscience* (Online). December 2014; 3(2).

[48] Hadhazy, A. Think Twice: How the Gut's "Second Brain" Influences Mood and Well-Being. *Scientific American*. February 12, 2010.

[49] Breus, M.J. Low on Vitamin D, Sleep Suffers. 2016, March. Retrieved from www.huffingtonpost.com.

Chapter 13: A Scientific and a Holistic View from the Hospital

[1] Wallace, J.B. Researchers Document Troubling Rise in Strokes in Young Adults. *The Washington Post*. May 11, 2016.

[2] Retrieved from www.strokeassociation.org

[3] Retrieved from www.strokeassociation.org

[4] Retrieved from www.cdc.gov.

[5] Retrieved from www.hsph.harvard.edu/news/press-releases/plant-based-diet-reduced-diabetes-risk-hu-satija/

[6] Red Meat Linked To Increased Risk of Type 2 Diabetes. 2011, August. Retrieved from www.hsph.harvard.edu.

[7] Red Meat Consumption Linked to Increased Risk of Total, Cardiovascular and Cancer Mortality. 2012, March. Retrieved from www.hsph.harvard.edu.

[8] Behall, K.M., Scholfield, D.J., Hallfrisch, J. Whole-Grain Diets Reduce Blood Pressure in Mildly Hypercholesterolemic Men and Women. *Journal of American Dietetic Association*. 2006, September; 106(9): 1445-1449.

[9] Low Vitamin D Predicts More Severe Strokes, Poor Health Post-Stroke. *American Heart Association News.* 2015, February.

[10] Whiteman, H. Vitamin D Deficiency Linked to Poor Brain Function, Death After Cardiac Arrest. 2014, October 19. Retrieved from www.medicalnewstoday.com.

[11] In Type 2 Diabetes, Vitamin D Deficiency May Play a Role in Hardened Arteries. 2014, September 21. Retrieved from www.vitamindcouncil.org.

[12] Yue, W., Xiang, L., Zhang, Y.J., et al. Association of serum 25-hydroxyvitamin D with symptoms of depression after 6 months in stroke patients. *Neurochemical Research* 2014; 39(11): 2218-24.

[13] Walk, Don't Run, Your Way to a Healthy Heart. 2013, April. Retrieved from www.heart.org.

[14] Regular Exercise Critical for Heart Health, Longevity. American College of Cardiology. *Science Daily.* 2016, January.

Chapter 15: Science for the Health of Caregivers

[1] Mario D. Garrett, M.D Caregiving: What Harm Can It Do? *Psychology Today.* 2013, March.

[2] Caregiving in the U.S. 2015. National Alliance for Caregiving. 2015, June. Retrieved from www.caregiving.org.

[3] Caregiver Statistics. Caregiving Action Network. Retrieved from www.caregiveraction.org.

[4] Ibid

[5] Hudson, Tori. Rhodiola: Stress, Fatigue, Mood, Reproductive Health. 2006, December. Retrieved from www.drtorihudson.com.

[6] De Bock, K., Ejinde, B., Ramakeers, M., Hespel, P. Acute *Rhodiola rosea* Intake Can Improve Endurance Exercise Performance. *Inter-*

national Journal of Sport Nutrition and Exercise Metabolism. 2004; 14: 292-301.

[7] Brown, R.P., Gerbarg, P.L., Ramazanov, Z. Rhodiola rosea: a phytomedicinal overview. *HerbalGram.* 2002; 56: 40-52.

[8] Darbinyan, V., Kteyan, A., Panossian, A., et al. Rhodiaol rosea in stress induced fatigue - a double blind cross-over study of a standardized extract SHR-5 with a repeated low-dose regimen on the mental performance of healthy physicians during night duty. Phytomedicine. 2000; 7(5): 365-71.

[9] Spasov, A.A., Wikman, G.K., Mandrikov, V.B., et al. A double-blind, placebo-controlled pilot study of the stimulating and adaptogenic effect of Rhodiola rosea SHR-5 extract on the fatigue of students caused by stress during an examination period with a repeated low-dose regimen. *Phytomedicine.* 2000; 7: 85–9.

[10] Panossian, A., Wikman, G., Sarris, J. Rosenroot (*Rhodiola rosea*): Traditional Use, Chemical Composition, Pharmacology and Clinical Efficacy. Phytomedicine. 2010, June; 17(7): 481-93.

[11] Gonzales, G.F., Villaorduna, L., Gasco, M., Rubio, J., Gonzales, C. Maca (Lepidium Meyenii) A Review of Its Biological Properties. *Revista Peruana de Medicina Experimental Y Sulud Publica.* 2014; 31(1): 100-10.

[12] Astragalus/University of Maryland School of Medicine. Retrieved from www.umm.edu.

[13] Astragalus/Memorial Sloan Kettering Cancer Center. Retrieved from www.mskcc.org.

[14] American Ginseng. U.S. National Library of Medicine. Retrieved from www.medlineplus.gov.

[15] Stamets, P. *Myco Medicinals: An Informational Treatise on Mushrooms.* Mycomedia Productions. Olympia, Washington. 3rd Edition. 2002.

[16] Ibid.

[17] Wu, X., Zeng, J., Hu, J., Liao, Q., Zhou, R., Zhang, P., Chen, Z. Hepatoprotective effects of aqueous extract from Linghi or Reishi mushroom Gandodrema lucidum (higher basidiomycetes) on amanitin-induces liver injury in mice. *International Journal of Medicinal Mushrooms.* ,2013; 15(4): 383-91.

[18] Batra P., Sharma, A.K., Khajuria, R. Probing Lingshi or Reishi Medicinal Mushroom Ganoderma lucidum (higher Basidiomycetes): A Bitter Mushroom with Amazing Health Benefits. *International Journal of Medicinal Mushrooms.* 2013;15(2): 127-43.

[19] Stamets. Ibid

[20] Ibid.

[21] Cohen, M.M. Tulsi – Ocimum Sanctum: a Herb for All Reasons. *Journal of Ayurveda Integrative Medicine.* 2014, October-December; 5(4): 251-259.

[22] Aranow, C. Vitamin D and the Immune System. *Journal of Investigative Medicine.* 2011, August; 59(6): 881-886.

[23] Cantorna, M., Snyder, L., Lin, Y.D., Yang, L. Vitamin D and 1,25 $(OH)_2D$ Regulation of T Cells. *Nutrients.* 2015, April; 7(4): 3011-3021.

[24] Vighi, G., Marcucci, F., Sensi, L., Cara, G., Frati, F. Allergy and the Gastrointestinal System. *Clinical and Experimental Immunology.* 2008, September; 153 (Supplement 1): 3-6.

[25] Caregiver Statistics. Caregiving Action Network. Retrieved from www.caregiveraction.org.

[26] Stiffelman, S. 14 Tips for Managing Anxiety After the Shootings. *Psychology Today.* December 2012.

[27] Conner, T.S., Brookie, K.L., Richardson, A.C., Polak, M.A. On Carrots and Curiosity: Eating Fruit and Vegetables Is Associated With Greater Flourishing in Daily Life. *British Journal of Health Psychology.* 2015, May; 20(2): 413-427.

[28] Shin, L.M., Liberson, I. The Neurocircuitry of Fear, Stress and Anxiety Disorders. *Neuropsychopharmacology.* 2010, January; 35(1): 169-191.

[29] Wieser, M.J., Butt, C.M., Mohajeri, M.H. Docosahexaenoic Acid and Cognition Throughout the Lifespan. *Nutrients.* 2016, February; 8(2): 99.

[30] Matsuoka, Y. Clearance of Fear Memory from Hippocampus Through Neurogenesis by Omega-3 Fatty Acids: A Novel Preventative Strategy for Posttraumatic Stress Disorder? *Biopsycholosocial Medicine.* 2011; 5:3. Online.

[31] Ullah, I., Park, H.Y., Kim, M.O. Anthocyanins Protect Against Acid-induced Excitotoxicity and Apoptosis via ROS-activated AMPK Pathway in Hippocampal Neurons. *CNS Neuroscience & Therapeutics.* 2013, November. Retrieved from www.onlinelibrary.wiley.com.

[32] Muchk, H. Magnesium and Affective Disorders. *Nutritional Neuroscience.* 2002, December; 5(6): 375-89.

[33] Foster, J.A., Neufeld, K.M. Gut-Brain Axis: How the Microbiome Influences Anxiety and Depression. *Trends in Neurosciences.* 2013, May; 36(5): 305-312.

[34] Smith, P.A. Can the Bacteria in Your Gut Explain Your Mood? *New York Times.* 2015, June 23. Retrieved from www.NYTimes.com.

[35] Messaoudi, M., Lalond, R., Violle, N., Javelof, H., et al. Assessment of psychotropic-like properties of a probiotic formula (*Lactobacillus helveticus* R0052 and *Bifidobacterium longum* RO175) in rats and human subject. *British Journal of Nutrition.* 2011; 105: 755-764.

[36] Bested, A., Logan, A., Selhub, E. Intestinal microbiota, probiotics and mental health: from Metchnikoff to modern advances: part III – convergence toward clinical trials. *Gut Pathogens.* 2013; 5:4.

[37] Ibid

CPSIA information can be obtained
at www.ICGtesting.com
Printed in the USA
FFHW01n0904240918
48532222-52424FF